BOYS — SEXUAL ABUSE AND TREATMENT

Rädda Barnen (Swedish Save the Children) works for children and young people based on the UN Convention on the Rights of the Child. We fight child abuse and exploitation and work for the protection of children in Sweden and all over the world. We provide assistance to these children and amass experience through practical action. We influence public opinion, values and attitudes in society through information and education.

Rädda Barnens Förlag publishes books for people who work with children in order to disseminate knowledge concerning the situation of children and provide guidance and impulses for new ideas and discussions.

ANDERS NYMAN AND BÖRJE SVENSSON

Boys – sexual abuse and treatment

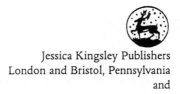

Jessica Kingsley Publishers
London and Bristol, Pennsylvania
and

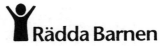

The right of Anders Nyman and Börje Svensson to be identified as authors of this work has been asserted by them in accordance with the Copyright, Designs and Patents Act 1988.

First Published by Rädda Barnen in 1995

First published in the United Kingdom in 1997 by
Jessica Kingsley Publishers Ltd
116 Pentonville Road
London N1 9JB, England
and
1900 Frost Road, Suite 101
Bristol, PA 19007, U S A

Copyright © 1997 Rädda Barnen and the authors
Editor: Dick Schyberg
Expert review: Lena Teurnell
English translation: Richard Nord Translations AB
Language review: Amy Brown
Graphic design: Stefan Lundström

Library of Congress Cataloging in Publication Data
A CIP catalogue record for this book is available from the Library of Congress

British Library Cataloguing in Publication Data
A CIP catalogue record for this book is available from the British Library

ISBN 1 85302 491 0

Printed and Bound in Great Britain by
Athenaeum Press, Gateshead, Tyne and Wear

Contents

Preface

Children should not be subjected to sexual abuse. This would appear obvious to most people, but unfortunately not to everyone. Article 34 of the UN Convention on the Rights of the Child states that children shall be protected "against all forms of sexual exploitation and sexual abuse" and that measures shall be taken to prevent "the exploitative use of children in prostitution" and "in pornographic performances and materials".

Rädda Barnen (Swedish Save the Children) has been deeply involved in the struggle against child sexual abuse since the late 1970s. We have featured the topic in seminars and publications and made it one of the common themes running through all our activities.

In 1990 we took the logical step of providing direct assistance to sexually abused boys by opening the Boys' Clinic. We wanted to amass as much knowledge and experience as possible so that we could develop effective methods and treatment models, but we also wanted to publicize the vulnerable situation of these boys. At that time there was a specialist clinic for sexually abused children in Stockholm. But almost all the children who came there were girls, who were treated by female therapists. As a result of a survey conducted by the Stockholm Department of Social Services, we knew that a large portion of sexually abused children are boys. That is why we decided to focus our efforts on them.

This book is a record of our work at the Boys' Clinic. The authors, Anders Nyman (psychologist) and Börje Svensson (social worker and psychotherapist) have been working on the project since the start. The programme has now been expanded by the addition to the staff of Margareta Eriksson (psychologist and psychotherapist), and the Boys' Clinic now also accepts a limited selection of girls for treatment, mainly sisters of boys already in therapy.

Our intention and our hope with this book is to guide and inspire others in their work with this group of abused children. "Making reality real" is the name of a chapter in the book. When it comes to sexual abuse, we all need to help to make this hard-to-fathom reality real so that we never close our eyes to the need for both preventive measures and help for these children.

STOCKHOLM, JANUARY 1995

LISA HELLSTRÖM
RÄDDA BARNEN

I. The phoney policeman

Patrik was ten years old and a city boy. He knew how to cross busy streets. On the way home from school he sometimes stopped and played in a park or went and looked in stores. He wasn't afraid, either of strangers or of cars. The world was a good place and he wasn't a shy boy. He trusted adults, and had no qualms about asking strangers for the time or directions. Nothing bad had ever happened to him.

One autumn day on his way home from school, Patrik was walking along a pedestrians-only street when suddenly a car came speeding along. Patrik never saw it and was hit by the car, which knocked him down and then drove off. Shocked and angry, Patrik got up and discovered that he had hurt his knee but was able to limp home. How could someone do that, hit and run, thought Patrik. First to drive on a street where traffic is prohibited, then to hit a child and leave the scene! Patrik wished he had seen the car's licence number. Then he could have reported it to the police.

The next day his knee was better. But on his mother's orders he went directly home from school. Not far from the door to his block of flats, a man was standing on the pavement. The man fixed his gaze on Patrik, and when he passed by the man opened his overcoat and showed a badge fastened to his jacket. The badge read POLICE in capital letters. Patrik stopped and asked:

"Are you a real policeman?"

"Yes," said the man.

Patrik immediately started telling the story of the hit and run

9

incident. The man listened and said:

"Where do you live?"

"I live in that building over there," said Patrik, pointing to a nearby doorway.

"If you show me the injury on your leg, I can tell who it was that hit you," said the man.

Patrik was happy that a policeman wanted to help him. At the man's suggestion, they went into Patrik's building to have a look at his injury.

Once inside the door, Patrik pulled up his trouser leg to show the man his injured knee. But the man didn't think that was good enough. He told Patrik to unbuckle his belt and pull down his trousers, as well as his underpants.

Suddenly Patrik got confused and frightened. But he pulled down his trousers. In an instant the nice policeman was transformed into a terrifying adult stranger. A scary grown-up who smelled of beer and was "icky". The man licked his finger and inserted it into Patrik's anus.

Now Patrik was scared to death. He didn't dare scream, since then the man might get angry and kill him. He probably had a knife in his pocket, thought Patrik. The man took out his penis and ordered Patrik to masturbate him.

Patrik smiled even though he was scared to death. He thought it was safest to look happy since then he might not get killed. Patrik smiled, but he couldn't help shutting his eyes and turning his head away. When Patrik had masturbated the man to ejaculation, the man put his hand in his pocket. Patrik was terrified. He thought the man was going to take out a knife and kill him. But instead of a knife, the man pulled a paper napkin out of his pocket, which he used to wipe his penis with.

The man threatened Patrik, saying that he would come back and get revenge if Patrik told anyone. Then he went away. Terrified, Patrik ran up the stairs to his flat.

When Patrik ran in through the door, both of his parents were home. He was holding his hands up in the air with his fingers spread out. No one was allowed to touch his hands. Patrik wanted desperately to wash his hands. He ran into the bathroom and rubbed his hands frenetically with soap. He continued washing and crying for a long time. His parents were perplexed. What had happened to the boy? When Patrik had finished washing he grabbed the cake of soap, ran into the kitchen and threw it into the garbage pail. He didn't want anyone else to use that cake of soap.

Then the dam burst. Weeping uncontrollably, Patrik fell into his mother's arms. When he had managed to tell them what had happened, his father ran down to the street to look for the man who had molested his boy. Soon he realized the search was futile and returned home. After an hour or so when the boy had calmed down a little, the family went to the police and reported the assault. Patrik was able to describe the perpetrator's appearance in detail: his face, the buckle on his belt, his shoes, what he smelled like and what accent he spoke with. The image of the perpetrator had etched itself into Patrik's retina and the odour of him remained in his organs of smell.

Thanks to the detailed description, the police were able to arrest the offender shortly after the assault. Unfortunately, however, he managed to molest another child, a seven-year-old, before he was arrested.

Patrik changed after the assault. He became timid and anxious, even though he tried to be like he was before. He was overwhelmed with fears. He laid kitchen knives beside his bed at night. He wanted to be armed in case his assailant should climb in through his window while he was in bed.

Patrik started sleeping in his mother's bed. He had nightmares about being abducted by strangers, locked in and murdered. When he woke up from these nightmares he lay thinking that maybe his assailant was on his way in through the window to kill him, or that he was hiding behind the shower curtain. The fact that Patrik lived on the fourth floor and that the perpetrator was now being held in detention by the police did not lessen his fear.

During the abusive act Patrik had shut his eyes and turned his head aside. This reaction now turned into a tic. Patrik couldn't stop blinking his eyes. His schoolmates asked him if he had got something in his eyes.

Patrik became extremely afraid of adult male strangers. When he walked along the street he took careful note of all men he encountered. When he saw someone he thought looked odd, he went out into the middle of the street or over to the other side to avoid meeting that particular man. When Patrik rode a bus or sat eating hamburgers with his mother, a strange man sitting nearby could trigger olfactory perceptions similar to those he had experienced during the assault. Then Patrik got frightened and had to change seats. His mother couldn't smell anything unusual.

Two weeks after the assault, Patrik came to the Rädda Barnen's Boys' Clinic for the first time.

2. Boys as victims

*P*atrik, *14 years old. Sexually abused by adult.* We started the Boys'
Clinic in Stockholm in the spring of 1990. With this heading on a
folder showing a picture of a lone boy leaning against a tree on the cover,
we tried to reach out to sexually abused boys with the message that they
now had somewhere to turn to get help.

As we look back five years later, we find that only two boys have
contacted us on their own initiative to talk about their problems. Both of
these boys wanted to be anonymous when they phoned, and neither of
them came to the Boys' Clinic. Many women writers have, in more or less
autobiographical accounts, described painful experiences of sexual abuse
to which they were subjected as children. Men have not written about
their experiences to the same extent or in such a manner that we have
been able to experience vicariously what it's like for a little boy to be
subjected to sexual abuse. One account of this kind that has come to our
knowledge is included in former boxer Bosse Högberg's memoirs Kontringen (1979), where he describes how he was forced to engage in a sexual
act by a girl several years his senior:

> *"Sit a little closer," she asked.*
>
> *I did, although I thought it was a little strange that we should sit
> that close together. Soon I felt her slender hand slip between my
> trouser legs.*
>
> *"What are you doing?"*
>
> *"Sit still, Bosse, don't be afraid," she whispered and grabbed my
> little cock.*

13

I felt it get hard. Like when I had to piss in the morning.

"I don't want to be with you," I said.

She pulled off my trousers. She lay down on her back and pulled me on top of her. With one hand she managed to get my little hard white worm in the crack between her legs.

"Don't be afraid, it's nothing dangerous," she said. And laughed.

I thought I would die.

"Let me go," I said.

She held me tight. I lay stock-still, paralyzed with fear. She lay still too.

"Let's have a look in the cook's shed," said someone on the street.

Vera pushed me off her and pulled up her trousers. I was shaking as if an electric current had passed through my body and managed to get my blue trousers on. Vera disappeared over the fence before I had both trouser legs on. She disgusted me. At night I couldn't get to sleep. I lay there staring at the ceiling, watching how the shadows danced and seemed to copulate. I heard her voice whisper over and over again until I thought I would go crazy. The whisper became a cry that echoed inside my head.

"It's nothing dangerous...it's nothing dangerous...it's nothing dangerous!" I had been involved in the most forbidden act in the whole world. And I was six going on seven. I felt waves of nausea in my stomach."

BOYS DON'T WANT TO BE VICTIMS

The example shows us how such an unpleasant memory can stay with us all the way into adulthood. Bosse Högberg is still in touch with the feelings of disgust and confusion he was left to deal with all on his own when he was a little boy.

Is the experience of being a victim so shameful for boys and so far from a traditional man's and boy's role that it cannot be described without risk to the victim's very sense of manhood?

Could it be that whenever possible, men and boys try to re-interpret a situation where they have been defenceless victims and turn it into a situation where they have themselves been active and responsible?

We came into contact with a man who had been sexually abusing his daughter for several years. In discussing the abuse he said:

"You have to understand, sex is so natural for me. It's something I've grown up with. Everyone was doing it when I was little, pulling at their dicks and making sexual gestures. I lost my virginity with a neighbour lady when I was seven."

What in our minds had been a clear case of sexual abuse had been defined by him as his sexual debut. He viewed himself as being precociously early in his sexual debut, rather than as a victim of child sexual abuse.

Another circumstance that is undoubtedly also a factor in explaining why boys remain silent about sexual abuse is the fact that most of the abusers are men. Many boys have expressed to us their concern at having been "infected" with homosexuality, or at the possibility that the perpetrator was in some way able to tell that the boy was "really a queer, deep down". This is particularly confusing if the sexual acts have in any respect also been associated with feelings of arousal and pleasure.

FIVE YEARS OF THERAPEUTIC WORK

In this book we have compiled some of the experiences we have had in our work with boys who have been victims of sexual abuse. We have had an opportunity to follow more than a hundred boys with varying histories of abuse in their struggle for vindication and security.

"Subjected to sexual abuse" is not a particularly useful diagnosis for therapy. Often it turns out that the sexual abuse is part of a larger psychosocial problem complex. Nonetheless, it is important to learn more about the particular areas that have to do with the sexual abuse, since it is there that the silence is most deafening.

This book summarizes five years of therapeutic work with over a hundred sexually abused boys aged 3–18 years.

The examples and case descriptions given in the book are camouflaged to make it impossible for outsiders to identify those involved.

The figure on the next page shows the relative proportions of sexual abuse inside and outside the family, and the relative proportions of different categories of abusers, for the boys we have had in therapy.

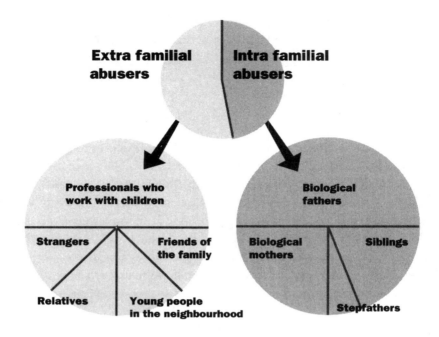

3. It started with a burn on the arm

— SEXUALLY ABUSED BY FATHER

Leo is five years old. When Leo's father was drunk he got sadistic and beat his mother. He had also hit Leo in front of his mother. But the mother didn't know that he had also abused the boy sexually.

One day she discovered a burn on Leo's arm. When she asked him how he got the burn, he replied he didn't know. Leo became evasive and withdrawn, didn't want to say anything. Knowing the father's violent disposition, the mother suspected that he may have been the one who deliberately burnt Leo. The mother became increasingly concerned about the boy's silence. A day or so later she said:

"But Leo, if you can't talk about how you got the burn you can at least make a drawing of how it happened."

To his mother's surprise, he did. On the drawing, Leo showed himself walking up to his father, who is sitting in a chair smoking. Leo drew himself several times to describe his movement towards the chair. When Leo gets to the chair, his father deliberately burns him with his cigarette.

The mother felt that making the drawing was a relief for Leo. Leo didn't want to comment on the drawing, but he said:

"Mummy, this isn't the worst thing that's happened."

"Do you want to draw some more?" his mother asked.

Leo nodded and made a new drawing. This one showed his father kicking Leo in the stomach. Leo repeated:

"Mummy, this isn't the worst thing that's happened."

His mother gave him a new piece of paper and Leo made another drawing. This time the picture showed his father touching Leo's penis.

Now Leo was revealing an incident of sexual abuse.

When Leo had drawn the picture he said that what the picture showed hadn't been an isolated incident, but had happened many times. Then Leo wanted to draw "many times".

Why was Leo able to draw what he couldn't describe in words? His father had forbidden him, under threat of punishment, to tell anyone about the sexual abuse. In the home there was a rock music poster with a skeleton. If Leo told anyone he would be as dead as the skeleton on the poster, his father had said. But he hadn't forbidden Leo to draw the incidents.

The knowledge that Leo's father had abused Leo sexually gave his mother the strength to separate and make the father move. After that she would not allow the father to have any contact whatsoever with Leo, nor did the father attempt to see his son. But she never dared to report the abuse to the police. The mother was afraid that he would come back and beat her to death.

During the time the abuse had occurred without the mother's knowledge, Leo had been self-destructive and had injured himself frequently. After Leo had disclosed the abuse and his father had moved it got worse. He banged his head against the wall, and tried to cut himself on kitchen knives. He often hurt himself. His mother constantly had to stop him from injuring himself.

He was like that for a whole year. Then he started directing his aggression towards his mother, punching and scratching her, screaming and threatening. Leo behaved in a sexually aggressive and provocative manner towards his mother, pulled down his trousers and masturbated in front of her. He yelled that he would "fuck" her and he tried to grab her between the legs when they were supposed to hug each other goodnight.

Leo came to the Boys' Clinic when he was seven years old. He ran around in the playroom, grabbed all the biscuits from the biscuit tray and stuffed them into his mouth. He took things out of his mother's purse and emptied her pillbox on the floor. He hit his mother on the back and burped in her ear. He used coarse, sexualized language unusual for a seven-year-old.

"Do you know what 'fuck you' means?" he said, using the English words.

"It means knulla dig," he replied to his own question.

"I got to suck my daddy's willy. Well, not his willy really, but that slimy thing that comes out when you pull it up."

Now he was able to describe the abuse in words. But without emotion, in an almost lustful tone, as if to shock or impress.

Approximately one-fourth of the boys who came to us have been sexually abused by their biological fathers. In many cases the sexual molestation is only part of a sadistic, tyrannical and capricious control that these fathers have exercised in their homes.

We have met boys who, besides the sexual episodes, have been tied up by their fathers, punched, threatened with a gun, held out of a window many storeys high and threatened with being dropped if they tell, forced to use oral snuff and drink alcohol, forced to watch violent and pornographic films or burnt and kicked in the stomach, as in the case described above.

EROTIC FORM OF HATRED

Who are these fathers who seem to be driven by a perverse need to torment their children?

Stoller (1986) defines perversion as "the erotic form of hatred". Perversion is a fantasy that is acted out. It is a sexual deviation whose foundation is hostility. By hostility, Stoller means a state where someone wants to harm another person. The pervert's hostility is formed in a fantasy of revenge. Concealed in fantasy and in the perverse acts is the original trauma. The function of revenge is to turn the trauma of childhood into triumph.

The rage that comes out of denied grief and denied emotions for an adult sexually abused as a child serves as a breeding ground for perversion.

Hedlund (1989) writes:

> In the sexually deviant act, rage is transformed into victory over the person or persons who made him unhappy. The trauma is turned into triumph. The vengeance creates sexual arousal. It is not just the actors in the drama who change places, the affects are also transformed into their opposites. The victim, who was helpless, vulnerable and defenceless, becomes the perpetrator, the one who controls, manages

and directs. As his tool he uses the part of his body that was the symbolic target of the attack on his sexual identity.

Because it is with his son that a father can identify most strongly, the son also becomes the one who gives the father the greatest opportunities for projection of repressed emotions. He unloads his feelings of self-hatred and powerlessness onto the child. The act of vengeance is directed towards the son, who through his very existence is a constant reminder to the father of his own childhood traumas. When the father physically abuses and sexually violates his child, he is striking against the repressed image of his own victimization.

Künstlicher (1991) writes:

> *If oppression and circumstances have deprived a person of the possibility of self-respect, that person becomes incapable of either feeling respect for his own integrity or showing consideration for the integrity of other people, something which in turn is inflicted on the defenceless child. Through his very defencelessness the child becomes a reminder of the violation which the adult does not want to acknowledge. And because he was never able to assimilate the humiliating experiences, the reminder must be wiped out. This is done by means of unconscious actions and attitudes, whose purpose is both to find an outlet for the feelings that are not recognized and to retain the unawareness. The child has to personify both the victim, through his powerlessness and his shortcomings, and the offender in order to fulfil his role in the unconscious drama. In this way the parent can direct all his contempt and all his hatred towards the child.*

CRUEL ACTS

Cruel acts spring from the need to avenge a real or imagined injustice (Lindbom-Jakobson and Lindgren 1994). When threatened with being put in an inferior position, the person who commits cruel acts attempts to assert his superiority towards others in order to enhance his self-esteem and ward off the threat of narcissistic violation. In order to preserve the narcissistic self-image of unlimited superiority, feelings of vulnerability in the abuser's own ego must be split off from his self-image and projected onto the victims. Primitive envy is an ever-present affect. To preserve his own omnipotent position under threat of fear and primitive envy, the perpetrator employs splitting-off and projection as a defence. By denigration of the victims he elevates himself to a position of power over their lives in order to evade the threat of inadequacy and inferiority himself.

DAD GOT A JANUS FACE

At the Boys' Clinic we sometimes come into contact with adult men who tell about how sexual abuse by their fathers has affected their lives. The following story comes from a 45-year-old man, Bertil, who has not had an opportunity to process his emotions surrounding his father's abuse of him:

> I was eight years old when the abuse began. My dad was an alcoholic. When he was drunk, one of two things could happen. If I was up, I got beaten for no reason. If I was in bed, I got sexually abused. Dad came into my room, lifted up the cover at my feet and started licking. He licked along my legs up into my crotch. I remember how I would lie rigid with fear, waiting for him to come into my room. I didn't dare show I was awake. As soon as he got near the bed I got as stiff as a stick. I blocked out all emotions. This went on until I was a teenager. Then my dad died.

The consequence of the abuse was that the boy's picture of his father was split into two.

"Dad got a Janus face."

On the one hand, Bertil's father was the person Bertil looked up to and loved, on the other hand he was an evil and terrifying devil who could make him rigid with fright and turn him into a stick.

During the period the abuse was going on, Bertil stopped believing in God. He thought that if daddy can let me down, so can God. There was no one to trust. When his father died, Bertil's mother grieved. Bertil didn't want to tell his mother what his father had done.

"She wouldn't have been able to take the truth."

Bertil grew up and devoted his life to taking care of his mother. His sisters and brothers got married and had children of their own. When Bertil was forty years old, his mother died. Then he got up the courage to tell his older sister, with whom he had shared a room as a small boy. He thought she might also have been abused or had maybe noticed what he had endured.

"But she didn't believe me, said that it was all in my imagination."

Bertil told us that he was now in a difficult situation. He didn't trust men, and believed women couldn't handle hearing difficult things. Bertil had been in therapy with a female therapist.

"She just put a lid on the whole mess."

Bertil had never had sexual relations with either men or women.

When Bertil was being sexually abused by his father, he turned himself into a non-person, an object, a "stick". As a shield against the confusion and pain, he withdrew his feelings. As an adult he continued doing the same thing. He withdrew from human intimacy and didn't trust other people.

4. Why did she do it?

"It was like I was two different people. Sometimes I just lost control. I knew it was wrong, but I couldn't stop myself."
This was how Martin's mother expressed how it felt for her when she sexually abused her son regularly during a six-year period. During the first three years of Martin's life, he lived at home with his mother and father. His mother acted out her mentally sick impulses with the boy. She sexualized her care of him, stroked his penis and encouraged him to stroke her genitals. She masturbated the baby and tried to perform intercourse with him. She smeared him with urine and faeces, which she allowed to dry. She isolated him from other children. During these three years, Martin was constantly harnessed to his pram or his push-chair when he was outdoors. He could scarcely walk and couldn't speak at all.

Due to the mental inadequacy of both his mother and his father, Martin was placed in a foster home when he was three years old.

No one suspected at the time that the boy was being sexually abused. Martin was placed in a religious foster home with authoritarian methods of child-rearing. He was often beaten and locked in as punishment. Every other weekend he went home to his mother and father. His mother continued molesting him, and his father pretended not to notice. When Martin was six and a half years old, the foster home didn't want him anymore. He was too difficult and was placed in a new home by the social services.

When Martin came to the new foster home he was frightened and destructive. He flung himself against doors, tried to jump off the balcony

23

and from windows. He took scissors and knives and said he was going to cut himself; sometimes he planned to cut off his penis. "I can take care of myself!" he screamed continually.

If people said something nice to him, he shrieked that they shouldn't lie. Martin hardly dared go to sleep, partly because of nightmares, and partly because he didn't want to close his eyes. He would lay in bed struggling to keep them open. When his foster mother gave him a shower, he refused to close his eyes when he was being shampooed. When he did manage to get to sleep, he dreamt that the whole bed was full of snakes. When his foster mother came in to console him, he got more scared of her than of the snakes. When she wasn't able to console him she took him into her bed. Then he got even more terrified and crawled over and hid himself behind his foster father's back.

Martin was unable to control his bowels. Every time his foster parents went to change him he would go wild and start masturbating compulsively. If his foster mother lay down on his bed to rest during the day, Martin would come up with a blanket and wrap her up in it. He was always very careful to wrap her arms in the blanket.

"I don't know what you do with your arms when you're sleeping," he would say.

When the foster family sat in the living room to watch television, Martin would sit in front of his foster mother with his legs apart and start to stroke his penis until he got an erection. Then he wanted his foster mother to touch herself between her legs.

The foster parents suspected that the boy had been sexually abused. But they didn't suspect his mother of being the perpetrator. They were more inclined to suspect that someone in the boy's former foster home had regularly molested him. The foster parents turned to the mother and told her of their suspicions. The mother then got it in her head that Martin had told the foster parents that she was the perpetrator. She therefore confessed, but not to everything at first. When the foster parents told Martin that his mother had admitted to abusing him sexually, he went crazy. He screamed:

"Why can she tell when I couldn't!"

Then he found out exactly what his mother had said and refused to say

anything more. But he revealed that more had happened by asking:
"Didn't she say anything else?"

SEXUALIZED CARE

Our experience is that sexual abuse by a woman is easier to conceal than sexual abuse by a man. Women's sexual abuse of boys can be masked by physical and emotional care of the child. It can often be difficult to draw the line between normal motherly physical care and intimacy, and more sexualized fondling. One boy told how his mother was always examining him to see if he had a hernia. Another boy was washed, powdered and made to wear nappies by his mother up to the age of around ten. A third mother wanted her son to examine her to see if she had threadworm in her rectum.

"These examinations would be made according to certain rituals, and it wasn't until I was an adult that I understood she actually got an orgasm from it."

A pre-pubescent boy who sleeps in his mother's bed doesn't arouse the suspicion of incest in others to the same degree as when a pre-pubescent girl sleeps in her father's bed. Allen (1990) relates a hypothesis put forward by Groth and Birnbaum: that when women are sexual abusers it is usually a question of incest, so the abuse is seldom reported. This hypothesis confirms our experience. In ten cases of boys who had been sexually abused by female abusers, the abuser in eight of the cases was the biological mother.

INVENTED OWN LANGUAGE

Peter remembers standing on a chair in the kitchen without any clothes on. His mother was also naked. She was big and stout. She hugged him and touched him all over his body and wanted him to touch her. He also remembers that there was food in the refrigerator and that he wasn't allowed to play out of her sight.

The memories are from a time when Peter was six years old and younger. His mother also often wanted to "cuddle" with him. They would lie naked in bed. His mother would touch his penis and he would touch her between the legs. Peter and his mother invented their own language, which no one else understood.

During this period the parents separated. The father moved away and the mother was given custody of Peter. The father's visitation rights were not respected by the mother. The mother didn't want Peter to see his father, and the father wasn't willing to fight for his visitation rights. The father remarried.

When Peter was six years old, the staff at his day nursery sounded the alarm. The abuse was revealed. The crime was considered to be verified by the evidence, but the prosecutor dropped the charges. The mother was judged to be unreceptive to either treatment or punishment. Peter moved in with his father and the father's new wife.

When Peter came to us he was a teenager. He said he hadn't told anyone about the abuse because he was a coward. Peter thought that people could see by looking at him that he had been sexually abused. He felt embarrassed when he changed clothes in gym. He said he found reading and arithmetic difficult, but was physically active. He liked outdoor life and scouting and playing with little children, "cuddling" with them. On several occasions he had sexualized his games with small children. Once he went off with a seven-year-old boy. He unbuttoned the boy's fly and pulled his penis. Peter also took out his own penis and wanted the seven-year-old to touch it. An adult came along and stopped the abuse. Peter's father and stepmother found out about the incident. Peter didn't think it was solely his fault, since the seven-year-old had come along willingly.

KISSED HIS MOTHER WITH AN OPEN MOUTH

When Stefan came to us he was eighteen years old, unemployed and living with his girlfriend. It was his girlfriend who persuaded him to come to the Boys' Clinic. She found out that Stefan used to kiss his mother with an open mouth.

Stefan had then begun to talk about his vague memories. He remembered his mother holding him tight, and that they didn't have any clothes on. Maybe he lay in his mother's bed. Her knee was in his crotch. Or was it her hand? He had difficulty remembering hands, especially his

26

mother's. He remembered that he wanted to have a pillow between his legs when he slept in his mother's bed, but couldn't remember why. He knew he had seen his mother masturbate in the toilet with the door open. He had also seen his father force her to have sex.

Maybe his mother was more attracted to Stefan than she was to her husband. He slept in the same room as his parents until he was fifteen years old. His mother often pestered him and wanted to kiss him with an open mouth. She tried to bribe him to give her "real" kisses.

"You can do better than that! That was no real kiss."

When the father saw how the mother was sexualizing her relationship with Stefan, he advised him to let her have her way.

"She needs it," his father said.

The mother was often depressed. Then she would take out a knife and say that Stefan was the one who decided whether she should live.

Stefan was a poor achiever in school with a great deal of absence and the lowest grades in the class. He was always thinking about his mother and whether he would be responsible if she committed suicide. When he felt particularly worried about his mother he skipped school and stayed home to make sure she didn't hurt herself.

When he came to us he had broken off contact with his parents. But he was still suffering from the effects of his mother's abuse. He couldn't stand it when his girlfriend hugged him. When they had sex he didn't want to be touched by her hands. Just to be sure, he held her arms pressed against the sheet. He couldn't enjoy sex. He felt like a robot, mechanical.

Stefan had fantasies of molesting children.

"Think if I were to hurt her," he had thought about a child at the day nursery where he had worked.

But he was frightened by these thoughts and pushed them out of his mind, wondering if he was normal.

ISOLATED BY SICK MOTHERS

The cases of sexual abuse by mothers with which we have come into contact have, as a rule, continued over a long period of time, often years. They started early in the child's life. The mothers were clearly mentally disturbed. None of the mothers had been sentenced to either prison or treatment for sexual offences, according to statistics from the National Prison and Probation Administration, which show that during the period 1986–92, an average of only two women per year were sentenced to prison for sexual offences. The children have not spontaneously reported the abuse. In every case, a concerned outsider has persuaded the child to tell.

The children have been isolated by their sick mothers. The fathers have either left the relationship or thought it best to let the mothers have their way. In many cases the fathers were afraid of these sick women. For some children, the sick world inside the home has become normal, while the healthy world outside the home has become abnormal.

Deviant and perverse behaviour can be a sign that the abused child misses his mother. Martin, the boy who was smeared with his mother's urine and faeces, had periods when he would smear toilet mirrors and walls with his own faeces. He would say:

"When I miss my mummy I play with poop."

The children we have met who have been victims of sexual abuse by their mothers have been confused and disoriented. Once they have gained a little perspective on the abuse, they constantly ask:

"Why did she do it?"

But the question is seldom put to the abuser. Loyalty and the child's yearning for a normal mother are strong, even after the child has been moved to a safe environment. Confronting the mother with this central question can mean being rejected.

5. Sibling incest

— AN UNEXPLORED FIELD

Sexual and physical abuse, molesting and violation of sexual boundaries within the family are not limited to offences committed by parents against their children. The offender may also be an older brother or sister.

We have in some cases come into contact with families where the children have engaged in sexual activities with each other in a way that is far beyond the realms of what can be considered normal and healthy exploration.

Little research has been done on the subject of inter-sibling sexuality. We don't know how common it is for siblings to engage in advanced sexual acts with each other.

There are, however, a number of descriptions in fictional literature, both of mutual sexuality and of what can be more accurately characterized as out-and-out abuse.

KAJ FÖLSTER

In her book *De tre löven* (1992), Kaj Fölster describes how her brother, who was nine years older, subjected her to all kinds of more or less abusive "experiments" during their childhood without any consideration of how painful they might be to his little sister. Some of the experiments were also sexual in nature:

> One day when we were at home alone he sat down in the big red armchair at the pewter table and ordered me to come to him. He told me to sit on his lap, higher and higher up. He talked about his penis

and whatever, and my whatever. He was going to teach me so much,
because he knew something girls like and need. Now he was going to
show me how it was done. He took off my panties without noticing how
I struggled against him. He held me firmly about the waist with one
hand while his other hand fondled my labia, and all the time he asked
me if I felt anything pleasant. He searched for "places" more and more
frantically.

I sat there petrified and just kept whispering "No" and "No" and
"No". I was awash in an ocean of fear and anxiety, a wish to die
engulfed in helplessness, with petrified emotions.

All of this is etched into my memory, even though I lost all sense of
time and don't know how I got away from him. But my attempts to
avoid repetitions succeeded. My own promise to never, never tell
anyone lay burning under my skin, everything else was pushed deeper
down.

SAM LIDMAN

In his memoirs entitled *Ett herrans liv* (1988), Sam Lidman describes how
he and his brothers and sisters engaged in sexual games:

Gradually the games became more advanced. One day Sven got an
idea, from where I don't know, since he was discreet. He lay down on
the bed in the back room with his arms over his eyes and said with a
loud voice: "Sven is dead now!"

A meaningless line for the uninitiated, but my sisters knew
precisely what he meant. Just as I now also realize how sophisticated
Sven must have been even then. From that time he was quite unaware
of what was happening to him, and completely guiltless. He neither
saw nor heard; everything was concentrated on feeling.

Bibi and Eva obediently went up to the bed and unbuttoned his fly
from either side, pulled down his trousers and underpants and began
stroking his organ, both of them, curiously and carefully until it finally
ejaculated.

The whimpers of pleasure escaping the corpse made me exceedingly
envious, and when he came I was close to dying myself of curiosity. It

would be couple of years before I got my first dose, up in a closet on a
lovely ledge together with Eva at Frejgatan 52 in the autumn of 1937.
(...)

I have never had the slightest qualms of conscience about these
games. They are among the nicest memories of my childhood. The only
thing I "regret" was that I wasn't allowed to be in on what happened
down by the tent. And although I went farther than my brother, and
my sisters showed me the greatest understanding, when the time came
for me as well I can nevertheless only feel sorry about the fact that I
was forced to keep things within the family so long.

ULF LUNDELL

In his novel *Saknaden* (1992), Ulf Lundell describes how the main
character Florian is initiated at the age of fourteen by his sixteen-year-old
sister on a summer meadow:

(...) and Anita unbuttoned my fly and I knew that what she was doing
was wrong because she was my sister but she was my big sister and she
wanted to show me something and I loved her so much and the grass
was tall and no one could see us and I heard her humming one of those
Beatles songs and then she tugged at my trousers and I lifted my body
and she managed to get my trousers and underpants down to my knees
and I looked again and she was straddling my thighs and smiling and
then she laughed and told me to close my eyes, I had to close my eyes
and I couldn't see anything, I closed my eyes again (...)

"Take it easy, little brother. Now I'm teaching you how to do this so
that you'll be able to do it too."

And she rode me slowly there in the grass and stroked me and
gave me light kisses until I started to thrust up into her and got my
arms around her and we embraced each other and we rolled around
so that I got on top of her and we lay there in the grass until she had
taught me what she wanted to teach me.

Two of the literary passages above describe sibling sexuality in an
emphatically positive tone. Fictitious or not, there is naturally no way for

us to know whether these sexual games were harmful or not.

But we do believe that experiences such as these between siblings are not everyday occurrences and could be understood as an acting-out of some kind of lack of boundaries within the family.

TWO TYPES OF SIBLING ABUSE

Pierce & Pierce (1990) say that sibling abuse can be divided into two categories. In the one case it is a matter of early, mutual exploration which stops when the children realize that they are doing something which they shouldn't be doing. In the other case it is a question of one sibling forcing another sibling to engage in sexual activities. In these cases the abuser is sometimes also being abused by a parent or relative.

From our experience at the Boys' Clinic we can identify two types of sexuality between siblings: symbiotic and sadistic. We choose to define symbiotic sexuality as abuse here as well, since in our experience it is usually a highly traumatic experience for both parties, even if there is no really aggressor but only two victims.

ALL WE HAD WAS EACH OTHER

Anette was the mother of six children with four different fathers. All six children were eventually taken into care and placed in foster homes. Anette lived only periodically with the fathers of her children. She had episodes of heavy drinking, during which times the flat was a den of drunks with different men wandering in and out. Some or all of her children also lived with her at different periods, depending on how she was managing her drinking problem at the time and how the children's different foster home stays were working out.

During one period, two of the children were living with Anette: Jessica, two years old, and Stefan, five. Andreas, seven, would come to stay with them for a weekend every now and then.

When he was eighteen, Stefan described this period as follows:

I remember how we children would sit close together under a table, not saying a word, watching mum sitting on the sofa with different men drinking booze. Sometimes they fought, sometimes they fucked and at least once I know she was raped. Sometimes we slept under the table, and when we woke up there may not be anyone there, and once a fire started in a mattress when we were alone and the door had been locked from the outside. Then we screamed until the neighbours phoned the fire brigade.

Sometimes we rode the metro at night. We were on our way to someone we didn't know. Mum dragged us along everywhere but didn't give a shit about us, all we had was each other.

Then I eventually wound up in a foster home, but I still went home to visit Anette sometimes. That was when everything started. I was ten years old and Jessica was seven. It was when Anette was living with Lennart and he was nuts. He put his cock up on the kitchen table and was going to give us some sexual instruction. He was always going on about sex with us and told me, for example, that I should be careful so I didn't get Jessica pregnant. I was only ten years old, I didn't under-stand anything about that stuff then.

But I do remember when Jessica pulled me into the toilet and wanted us to hug. She showed me how you were supposed to do it. She held me hard and pressed her whole body against me and wanted us to kiss "grown-up kisses". She said we should also moan like grown-ups, "uh, uh, uh, uh", when we hugged. I'm sure she must have seen Anette and Lennart or that Lennart must have been at her.

We used to do that when I came to visit, as a game that just continued. It got to be more and more, and at the end when I was sixteen and she was thirteen we lay on top of each other with our trousers down and sort of humped. She touched me but I didn't dare touch her. We didn't really have sex, but I'm sure that if we had continued we would have, since it kept getting more and more advanced.

It usually followed the same pattern every time. It was always when we were alone. We might just look at each other in a certain way, or one of us might kid around with the other by sticking out a foot or throwing a pillow, always with that look that put us in a certain kind of mood. Then we might chase each other or have a pillow fight or wrestle and sort of touch each other and then we started unbuttoning

each other's clothes. It ended with someone not wanting to do it
anymore and we would like get upset and angry with each other. Then
I might call her a "whore" or she might say "fucking queer" to me.

THE INNER BOUNDARY

From the very start, children have a need for protection, warmth and physical contact. Children enjoy caressing. There are no inborn taboos as to what parts of a child's body we are "permitted" to touch. The only thing the child perceives is that touch feels different on different places on the body: it tickles, feels warm, is more intense, or less intense.

It is adults who show the child where on the body touch is permitted and in what manner. An inner perception of a boundary is sensed where the adult's hand stops caressing. But when the hand fails to define this boundary, either by overstepping it or by not caressing the child at all, how is the child has to know where the boundary is? When children are left to themselves, neglected, abandoned or violated, when they have been forced to turn to each other for closeness, protection and warmth, how are they then supposed to develop a sense of what is permitted and what is not?

We believe this is what happened in Stefan and Jessica's case. The children had only each other to turn to in traumatic situations. They lived in an environment where sexual and physical boundaries were constantly overstepped, which contributed towards the sexualization of their needs for closeness and physical contact. They developed an emotional dependence on each other in lieu of a natural relationship with an adult.

THE HANSEL-AND-GRETEL SYNDROME

Such a relationship between siblings is usually referred to as the "Hansel-and-Gretel Syndrome" (Furniss 1991). The fairy-tale of Hansel and Gretel is of course about two small children who are left in the forest by their father to fend for themselves and are unable to find their way back. They are two abandoned children who depend on each other for survival, comfort and protection.

When it comes to the Hansel-and-Gretel syndrome, it is therapeutically meaningless to single out either an abuser or a victim. Both children are

34

acting out the neglect and the physical and mental abuse to which they have been subjected. Even if it often appears from the outside as if the boy has been the active party and the girl the passive one, the boy cannot be treated as if he were an adult offender. This only makes him a scapegoat. The mutual dependence between such children has quite a different dynamic than that between an adult abuser and his victim.

Nevertheless, the girl in such a situation risks developing the same symptoms in the form of sexualized behaviour and thereby runs the risk of being abused in the future, just as is the case with other exploited children.

The boy is also at risk of developing an abuser behaviour if he does not get the help he needs. Brothers and sisters who use each other in this way are lost children and need help from adults to find their way home again.

SADISTIC ABUSE

The dynamic is a different one in cases of more sadistic abuse. Here there is an identified offender and a helpless victim.

At the Boys' Clinic we have met Max, fourteen years old, and his little brother Robert, eight. Robert came one day to his mother and asked her what the slimy cream was that came out of Max's willy. It took a while for his mother to understand the implications of Robert's question, but eventually the whole story came out.

For as long as Robert could remember, Max had subjected him to experiments. He had forced Robert to drink urine, shoved him in the water where it was over his head to see what he would do when he couldn't swim, blocked the door to the sauna when it was on and Robert was in it to see how long it would take for him to panic, and so on.

The experiments were naturally frightening, and there was a compulsive repetition, almost a ritual characteristic to their performance.

Gradually the experiments also became sexual in nature. Max had read about oral sex in a magazine. He wanted to try it on Robert. Then he saw a television programme about anal sex and wanted to try that too. Max threatened to beat up Robert if he told anyone.

Max and Robert's parents were both highly educated, had high positions and worked a great deal. The boys attended private school. The

35

parents expected the boys to have excellent academic results, good behaviour and manners, a spotless appearance and success in sports. But they neither took the time nor were capable of seeing how the boys were really doing. And they had not discovered Max's systematic oppression of Robert.

Max was the brother for whom the parents had the highest expectations. At the same time he was the one who find it toughest to live up to them. When he failed to make the grade, he was sometimes subjected to corporal punishment by his father.

The father could not abide the boys' whining, crying or behaving like "sissies", or displaying any signs of weakness or dependency. On such occasions he was careful to point out that such behaviour would certainly not get them far in any field.

When we got the two brothers in therapy, we found that Robert was severely traumatized by his big brother's maltreatment of him and furious at his parents who had failed to realize what was going on. Max was being subjected to severe bullying in his school and suffered greatly under the burden of his parents', especially his father's, expectations.

Max had trained himself from an early age to hold back his emotions, both his tears and his rage.

He was good at both golf and tennis. It was important never to show your feelings when you lost or hit the ball out of bounds, he explained to us.

"If I played with daddy and got mad at something that happened in the game, he would just walk out."

As a result of this kind of upbringing, Max had become detached from his own emotions. Everything that had to do with feelings, impulses and drives was viewed by him as chaotic, abhorrent and unacceptable, something he couldn't cope with.

The abuse of Robert can be seen as an attempt to compensate for the powerlessness he experienced in his relationship with his father and the bullying he was subjected to in school. At the same time he used his little brother as a kind of "dustbin" for his fantasies, his impulses and his forbidden emotional life.

At first, Max found it very difficult to remember anything about the

36

abuse. He did not have "the foggiest notion" of how things had got this far or where he had got his ideas from. Moreover, he claimed that Robert was complicit in the behaviour and even almost an instigator of it.

"He thought it was fun, it was only a lark," said Max.

But what Max did with Robert was not a manifestation of normal curiosity or the urge to experiment. In our opinion, Max was at risk of repeating the abuse on others. It was important to draw attention to this, since he exhibited such a complete abuser personality.

His difficulties remembering, his tendencies to lay the blame on Robert, his denial and his complete lack of empathy with Robert's situation and feelings, combined with detachment from his own emotions, were clear signs.

Max needed to be supervised and checked whenever he was in the company of small children, and he needed treatment.

Robert perceived himself as "wicked and disgusting". Instead of asking girls in school if they wanted to "go steady" he would say: "Do you want to suck my cock?" Unlike Max, however, he was in touch with his pain and his fear and was able to express in words what it felt like when Max was cruel to him, which also proved crucial for his rehabilitation.

6. Refusing to grow up

— ABOUT PAEDOPHILES

The word "paedophile" comes from the Greek and is a combination of the words for child and love: paedo and philia – child love.

The paedophile's child love is based on a sexual desire for children who have not yet reached puberty and a sexual inadequacy and/or lack of desire when it comes to adults of the same age (O'Grady 1992). The paedophile is emotionally and sexually fixated on children. He, or sometimes she, has become stuck in a perversion which is often impossible to escape. The reason the sexual fixation on children is difficult to alter is, according to Hertoft (1977), that the perversion conceals anxiety-laden memories that must remain unconscious to prevent an emotional crisis. According to Glasser (1988), these anxiety-laden memories are of such a nature that they could precipitate a psychosis if they were not split off from the conscious mind.

There are adults who feel a sexual attraction towards children who do not seek to satisfy their craving in the form of sexual abuse. Martens (1991) presents Finkelhor's hypothetical model of the conditions that must be fulfilled for a potential offender to sexually molest a child:

1. He must find emotional satisfaction in being with children.

2. He must feel a sexual attraction to children.

3. He feels too inhibited to develop a deep and lasting relationship with an adult partner.

4. His natural inhibitions against initiating sexual liaisons with children must be broken down.

It is these natural inhibitions that determine whether the paedophile will become criminal or not. For example, the fear of punishment and the fear that the deviant sexual orientation will become exposed among family, friends and co-workers can be deterrent factors.

TWO TYPES OF PAEDOPHILES

Martens (1991) cites Groth, who differentiates between two types of paedophiles: the "regressed" and the "fixated".

The sexuality of the regressed paedophile is primarily directed towards adult partners. But in situations where he is exposed to stress and feelings of inadequacy, he turns his sexual desire towards children. Under harmonious and ordered family conditions, the regressed paedophile can have a normal sex life. But when he suffers a crisis and his emotional life becomes unbalanced, he is not sufficiently mature to solve conflicts, instead resorting to sexual acts with children as solace.

The fixated paedophile's sexuality is primarily directed towards children. The paedophilic orientation begins during adolescence. The sexual interest in children is not triggered by any particular conflicts or crises, but is permanent and stable. The fixated paedophile identifies with children and perceives himself as being on the same level as them. He has little or no sexual contact with peers, and is often single or married for the sake of appearances. When we at the Boys' Clinic talk about paedophiles, we mean fixated paedophiles.

Glasser develops this in a slightly different fashion. Instead of fixated paedophiles, he talks about "primary paedophilia", which is a perverse mental structure that helps the ego to remain relatively integrated and stable. Based on primarily paedophilia, Glasser makes a subdivision into "invariant" and "pseudoneurotic" personalities.

The invariant paedophile is an individual who has always been consistently sexually involved with children and/or adolescents, boys more often than girls. He has no sexual, and often no social, interest in adults, whether men or women. He can be characterized as a rigid

40

personality with a limited range of interests and activities. He displays no genuine guilt or shame over his paedophilia.

The pseudoneurotic paedophile may appear to be a normal, adult-oriented individual, although with occasional difficulties that may manifest themselves in impotence, sexual apathy and some tension and distress in his relationship with his partner. On superficial observation, these difficulties may appear to be neurotic.

Now and then he acts out his paedophilic urges, for which he feels great shame. But on the inside he is basically paedophilic. The paedophilic impulses persist below the surface of a "normal" sexuality. Potency in adult sexual relations is often stimulated by fantasies about sex with children during intercourse with an adult partner. Although the pseudoneurotic paedophile gives the superficial impression of being fundamentally different from the invariant paedophile, he is a profoundly disturbed individual.

AGGRESSION BELOW THE SURFACE

Both the invariant and the pseudoneurotic paedophile has an internal image of himself as a child, according to Glasser. He is in secret a violated child, who tries to get rid of his vulnerability and his rage by idealizing children and projecting his own sexual needs onto them. The idealization and the projections are fragile protective mechanisms that are always at risk of collapsing.

When the paedophile's sexual encounters with children become violent, this can naturally be interpreted in part as an attack on the hated parent, and in part as an attack on unwanted and shameful parts of the paedophile's own self, including a forbidden wish to be a girl, says Glasser.

There are fundamental similarities between sexual and physical abuse of children. The aggression is always there below the surface, even during the "gentlest" forms of molestation.

The paedophile acts out his sexuality towards children as if the child were capable of being an equal sexual partner. The paedophile tries to deny the differences between the generations and his own adulthood so that he can retain an omnipotent, grandiose self-image. According to Glasser, who also refers to Chasseguet-Smirgel and McDougall, this is the very foundation of the psychopathology of paedophilia. When the paedophile denies the differences between himself as an adult and the little child, it also becomes obvious to him that the child has the same sexual needs as he has.

More than forty percent of the boys we have treated at the Boys' Clinic have been sexually molested by unrelated persons. Nearly all of these children have been molested by paedophiles. Most of these children have been abused by persons whose profession has involved working with children: youth recreation leaders, day nursery staff, teachers, ministers, foster fathers, club leaders, fathers in back-up families, etc.

ORGANIZED PAEDOPHILES

Many paedophiles are organized in more or less clandestine associations which, among other services, provide addresses to places and individuals associated with the child sex trade. The North American Man/Boy Love Association (NAMBLA) is one such organization whose goal is:

> To organize support for boys and men who have or desire consensual sexual and emotional relationships and to educate society on their positive nature.

Another organization is the Rene Guyon Society (RGS). Their motto is:

> Sex before eight or else it's too late.

The organization had about 5,000 members, both male and female, in 1990. A paedophilic magazine called Børnebanden is distributed in Denmark.

The paedophilic culture promotes the view that sex between children and adults is not harmful to the children. They believe society causes harm to the children by bringing their paedophilic friends to court and punishing them.

The paedophilic subculture strengthens the "us against them" feeling and the illusion of being normal. It is as if there were a country – "Paedophilia" – where the paedophile is a normal, respected citizen surrounded by hostile, intolerant neighbours.

An extensive trade with child-pornographic films flourishes among paedophiles. More than three hundred hours of child-pornographic video-tape was confiscated from the "Huddinge sex ring" (a paedophilic sex ring uncovered in Huddinge, a suburb just south of Stockholm) in 1992. At least as much was confiscated by the police in Norrköping, a town about 160 km south of Stockholm, in the beginning of 1994.

In connection with these confiscations, a Swedish sect called Vi fria ("We Free") was also discovered, in which some eighty paedophiles had mutual contact via newsletters. These newsletters contained stories of sexual encounters with children plus ads asking for sexual liaisons with children. Here are some examples of such ads:

> *Entrust your daughters to me when you want to be on your own, for example when you go away on holiday. I will care for them gently and lovingly in every way. Suitable ages: around eight-nine years.*

> *Family with two daughters seeks other family. Our preference (not a requirement) is a family with one or more sons.*

> *Attractive man, 33 years of age, 181 cm/75 kg, fairly dark, seeks various Lolita types, but above all I wish to meet young women and children who like to masturbate.*

In a later issue the editorial staff issues a warning to the readers:

> *After a tip from a member we have discussed a complete revamping of the personal ads. There may be problems if the association arranges liaisons with minors. For this reason all ads in the future must be free of any reference to sex. An example of an ad is as follows: "I am thirty-three years old and wish to make contact with families. My interests are growing roses and building with lego."*

The Huddinge sex ring increased public awareness of the scope of the child-pornographic film industry and exactly what these films contain.

43

Every film depicts actual sexual abuse of one or more children. Children who have been forced to participate in such films can testify as to how violated they have been. The very knowledge that the films may be spread to a wider circle causes mental suffering:

"When I think about others sitting there watching me, I don't want to live," says the refugee boy Ben, 14 years old. He had been videotaped while being brutally beaten and raped at a police station in his homeland before he fled to Sweden.

Another way to spread pornographic pictures and film sequences is via computers linked to the Internet. Child pornography is stored in secret databases and can be downloaded by interested users.

EXPERTS AT MAKING CONTACT WITH CHILDREN

Just as the drug addict seeks out places where drugs are easily accessible, so the paedophile seeks out settings and professions where opportunities for natural contacts with children are great. Paedophiles become experts at contacting children, at being gently persuasive without using force, at gradually winning their confidence by taking a personal interest or through gifts.

Over the years we have had a number of sex rings in Sweden where paedophiles have abused boys in a residential area, a school or a club.

In raids the police have found hundreds of photographs of boys' penises and videotapes where the offender has filmed himself sexually abusing children. It is not unusual for paedophiles to keep their own card indexes with ratings of the children they have molested.

In a raid on the premises of a 36-year-old physical education teacher who had sexually abused numerous small boys, the police found a card index with a description of each boy:

Carl, 9 years old. Small, fair, soft boy with cute ass.

In some cases the index cards contained catalogued pubic hair cuttings or scrapings from the boy's anus.

44

There are examples of paedophiles who have abused hundreds of children. In an article entitled The treatment and rehabilitation of sexual offenders from 1946, Fairbairn (1952) reflects on the question of whether it is possible to treat sexual perversions with psychotherapy. Even though the article is nearly fifty years old, we think its arguments are valid today.

Fairbairn polemizes against those who consider sexual perversions to be an expression of a psychoneurotic problem complex. He believes that the neurotic personality differs from the perverse personality. The neurotic uses his psychological defence mechanisms to repress deviant sexual urges. It is only when the defences aren't adequate that perverse transgressions can occur, leading to strong feelings of guilt.

In the sexual pervert, by contrast, the perversion is not inhibited by the ego's defence mechanisms. The psychoneurotic defences have failed, and instead the pervert "capitalizes" his perverse tendencies instead of repressing them, with the consequence that they not only become overt, but assume a dominant position in the structure of his personality. "The resulting situation may, to use psychiatric terms, be summarized in the statement that the sexual pervert is not a psychoneurotic, but a psychopath," says Fairbairn.

If the sexual interest in children has come to dominate the entire personality, and shame and guilt are not effective restraining mechanisms, then we can better understand the paedophile's great sexual hunger for children. The sects, the magazines, the newsletters, the pornographic pictures are "capital" which is nurtured and multiplies.

Fairbairn did not believe it was possible to treat sexual offenders so that they are "cured" of their perversion. He did, on the other hand, have good personal experience of getting paedophiles to refrain from continued assaults on children. This could be accomplished through threats of punishment or through stricter requirements that they quite simply not be allowed to be around children. But also by teaching them to act out their perversion without direct contact with children. He didn't believe it was possible to eliminate the deviant sexual urge.

7. **I meant well**

— A LETTER FROM A PAEDOPHILE

Ron had committed sexual offences on a group of boys aged 10 to 13 for several years. Now he was in prison. He was a youth recreation leader and a sports instructor in a community in southern Sweden. Through his profession he came into contact with a large number of children in a "natural" way. It was a position of trust which, in the eyes of the community, he had violated and abused. But how did he view his own behaviour? A letter he wrote to the parents of the children gives us some insight into how a paedophile can reason about his own role in the lives of the children he has sexually abused.

This is what Ron wrote:

All I lived for was to give these children the benefit of everything I had developed and learned. To give them a secure and solid foundation for their future. The truth is that they sought me out because of all the rich and fine things we could share. Sexually it was never my intention to create anything that upset them.

It is also a fact that they had great trust in me as a warm and dependable human being. They often, both young and old, shared their personal and family troubles with me. To be able to truly understand this, you have to know the kind of person I really am and you have to have had close contact with the children and the positive involvement in sports we shared. Since I have also had long experience of people turning to me in times of trouble, I was able to help the children by explaining and many times straightening out difficult problems. The

47

gratitude and joy I received in return from both the children and their families gave me a great deal of strength and happiness.

Once again I would like to underscore the fact that it has **never** been my intention to hurt anyone. That I have always in all ways worked and acted on behalf of the children's future and best interests. Always taken responsibility for the mistakes I have made, and always in consultation with the children. Furthermore, I have always been desirous of improving myself and everything that isn't good, whether in me or in someone else.

I am writing to you now because I will soon be released. I have thought a great deal about how you and the children are doing and what you think about what happened and about me.

I am deeply unhappy about what happened. My feeling and my desire has always been to be a giving and supportive adult for your children. For this reason it has always been very painful, and so much was allowed to happen that wasn't good for either them or me. Things that should never have existed in my contact with the children. I never meant to hurt anyone, but many unfortunate circumstances have been at the basis of what happened.

I have served my sentence and I am working with myself. It now remains to be seen whether I am capable of coping with all the difficulties that await me when I get out. But I do not wish to cause any worry for you or your children now when I try to return to a normal life and parts of my career. I will not look up any of you myself. But if we should happen to run into each other somewhere and you clearly indicate that you want to stop and talk, I will be eternally grateful.

If any or all of you should wish to meet me to ask about anything or express what you think and feel, I will always take the time for this; in the very best way for everyone.

I hope that all the good things that we had can live on in all of you. For me, it is the only thing that has given me the strength to get this far.

At the trial, everything was lumped together in a disgusting mess and presented.

I always wanted to give every one of them as much as I could from

all I had experienced myself. To give them many fine building blocks
to build their future with. I can't help that this was my great joy. I
received a lot of positive and strong support from you parents. But at
the same time I betrayed the trust you placed in me. This is something
I will never get over. Something that I wanted to come to terms with in
private long before as well.

> *Thank you for everything that we struggled to achieve together.*
The support you all gave me. Something I will always carry within me.
I was very alone and gave everything I believed in for the children.
And yet it turned out so wrong.

COMMENTS ON THE LETTER

The picture Ron paints of himself is a picture of a warm and caring person. A grown-up friend who is understanding and helpful, both in sports training and with family problems. A human being who realizes that he has made some mistakes, but who seems to believe that the positive side of the children's relationship with him outweighs the negative side. He has lived for these children and feels that he has been unfairly treated. He has committed sexual offences without meaning to hurt anyone. He has never used violence. And the children did come to him, after all.

Why did Ron abuse the boys when he knew that what he was doing was wrong? He couldn't resist his own urges. His internal restraints against initiating sexual encounters with children had been broken. When Ron talks about the abuse, he is no longer a subject who bears responsibility for what he has done. Since his sexual urges were directed towards small boys, and since he also meant well towards them, he has to blind himself to the fact that the acts were harmful to them. He does this by pretending there are no differences between himself and the boys. Inside he doesn't experience the abuse as being harmful. Some harm may have been done when it was discovered. That was when the prosecutor described the incidents without presenting them in a positive context, so they were "lumped together in a disgusting mess". He loved the boys and their bodies. The sexual abuse was something that happened to occur when he "lived to give these children a secure and solid foundation for their future."

49

"It was never my intention to create anything that upset them."

No, he didn't wish to upset them. But he wanted to have sex with them.

Ron also implies that he tried to come to terms with something in private. But he isn't able to come out and say what it is. He doesn't take responsibility for the abuse by naming it. He wants to appear to be someone who meant well. "And yet it turned out so wrong."

The abuse is something that just "happens". There is nothing in the letter to indicate that he has been able to put himself in the children's place and understand what it has been like for them to have been sexually abused by him. He wants to see the bright side and "all the fine building blocks" he has contributed for the boys' future. He wants to clear things up so the parents will stop being angry with him. The sexual abuse has to be erased. He is full of his interest for the children, not just their sports but also their troubles and their joys. He cannot bear the picture of himself as being evil towards the children. The good must be made visible. The "disgusting mess" with which he was confronted in court is a threat to his self-image. He is struggling to avoid having to acknowledge the paedophilic sexuality that was a part of his involvement with the children.

The boys identified with him to some extent. He was their instructor and perhaps a role model. There is no reason to paint an entirely black picture of such a man, since the black paint may then taint the boys' own self-image. "What kind of person am I who could like such a horrible person?"

No, this man does not seem to have been an evil person. But he had a dangerous problem: he wanted to have sex with children. And in our judgement he will continue to want to have sex with children. The letter displays a lack of self-insight, which, in combination with an inability to empathize with the children's situation, to see things from their point of view, makes him a risk individual. There are no victims in the land of Paedophilia.

50

8. If you scream I'll kill you

We have only come into contact with four cases at the Boys' Clinic where the perpetrator has been a complete stranger to the victim and his family: A five-year-old boy who was raped at a refugee camp, a seven-year-old and a ten-year-old who were sexually assaulted in the stairways of their apartment buildings, and an eight-year-old who was raped while collecting empty cans in a park.

Of these four assaults, three were very severe and one was less severe. All four victims were deathly terrified at the time of the assault. The terror resulted in post-traumatic distress symptoms.

Does the fact that only a relatively small number of children treated at the Boys' Clinic were sexually abused by strangers mean that these offences are rare, but as a rule severe and frightening in nature?

The National Council for Crime Prevention (Martens 1990) investigated 886 cases of sexual abuse of children. 325 of these children were abused by an adult stranger.

In the group of children who had been abused by adult strangers, 2 percent had been subjected to consummated intercourse, 1 percent to attempted intercourse and 5 percent to oral sex. Fully 41 percent had reported "verbal sex", in other words sexual molestation in the form of sexually coloured and intimate questions or statements.

In the group of children who had been abused by adult acquaintances, 6 percent had been subjected to consummated intercourse, 5 percent to attempted intercourse and 12 percent to oral sex, while 30 percent had reported verbal sex.

In the group of children who had been abused by their fathers, 12 percent had been subjected to consummated intercourse, 11 percent to attempted intercourse and 16 percent to oral sex, while 13 percent had reported verbal sex.

According to the National Council for Crime Prevention, the mildest form of sexual offence against children is one committed by an adult stranger. The offences in this category are characterized by the fact that they are almost always of a non-recurring nature. They usually occur in a public place. A relatively large percentage of the victims are schoolboys. It is nearly equally common for the victim to be alone as to be together with another child of the same age in the abuse situation. In many cases, there is no direct physical contact with the victim. More than half of the reported perpetrators are not identified by the police. Verbal sex and sexual gestures with the body on the part of the perpetrator are the most commonly occurring acts. Of the cases with physical contact, fondling of intimate parts and sexual kisses, caresses and hugs are the most common forms. Physical violence is rare, but there is some element of compulsion. Permanent physical and mental injuries as a consequence of such abuse are relatively rare in this form of crime.

The study by the National Council for Crime Prevention also shows that sexual offences committed by acquaintances of the victim were more common than offences committed by strangers. The risk of being sexually abused in the home by a close relative or acquaintance is thus greater than the risk of being sexually abused by an adult stranger. Furthermore, the sexual offences when the perpetrator is an acquaintance of the victim are more severe than those where he is a stranger. The more closely acquainted the perpetrator is with the victim, the more severe the abuse.

Does this mean that we have reason to be less concerned about what "dirty old men" might do to our children? The following description of a case of sexual abuse of a five-year-old shows that there can sometimes be a very fine line between sexual molestation and murder by a stranger. The source of the story is a judgement rendered by the court of appeals.

SEVEN DOLLARS FOR INTERCOURSE
Eckard was a young man around twenty years old. He worked as a park

52

caretaker. The year before the aggravated rape of the five-year-old girl, he had molested a seven-year-old girl a number of times. On the first occasion, Eckard had offered the girl fifty kronor, or about seven dollars, for intercourse and then lured her into a storeroom in the basement of the building. On the second occasion he had followed the girl and offered her the same sum for intercourse. On the third occasion, when the girl was waiting for her mother outside the laundry room, Eckard had once again offered the girl seven dollars for intercourse. On each occasion the girl had become frightened and run away.

When Eckard was eventually questioned by the police, he admitted that he had frequently asked children if they wanted to have sexual intercourse with him. Eckard said he never meant the questions seriously. It was mostly just a joke.

Eckard was clearly an individual who got sexually excited by asking small children if they wanted to have intercourse with him. He had never crossed the threshold from words to action.

The worst act of violence he had ever committed was when he asked an eleven-year-old girl if she wanted to have intercourse with him. He offered the girl twenty kronor, or about three dollars. When the girl turned him down he shoved her into a snowdrift.

One overcast summer day the same year Eckard pushed the eleven-year-old girl into the snowdrift, he discovered five-year-old Lisa playing in her yard with several other children.

According to Lisa, a "boy" came up to her and asked her if she could show him the way to the public bathing beach, which was a short distance from Lisa's home. Lisa left her friends and accompanied Eckard, lured by the promise that he would give her some candy if she helped him. They walked towards the beach, but after a while they turned off the path and entered a wooded area. When they got to a rocky area, Lisa was tired and Eckard carried her past the rocks. Eckard asked if she wanted to have intercourse and Lisa replied yes, since she thought it had something to do with candy. Eckard put her down and they followed a small path into a densely wooded area. The place was not visible from the path or from the nearby residential buildings.

Now Lisa had to pee. Eckard first pulled down her pants, then his own

53

and exposed his penis. He tried to penetrate her. It hurt and Lisa, who was lying on a steep slope, became frightened. She started screaming that she wanted to go home. Eckard placed his hand over her mouth, put his hands around her throat and said:

"If you scream I'll kill you!"

Lisa couldn't breathe. She thought she was going to die. Suddenly Eckard released his stranglehold and walked away. Lisa walked back to the path on which they had come. On the way she met a woman. The woman saw Lisa walking and crying, with the back of her clothing all soiled. The woman stopped and asked her if she was alright. Lisa answered that a boy had tried to strangle her.

The subsequent medical examination found several discoloured skin areas and abrasions on Lisa's neck. There were red abrasions on her back between her shoulder blades and her neck. Between her shoulder blades there were bluish-red bands.

The injuries indicated that Lisa had been subjected to a stranglehold and that she had been dragged or had slid on her back. There were numerous haemorrhages in her face, around her eyes, on the upper parts of her neck and in her eyes. The haemorrhages revealed that the stranglehold had been so tight that the flow of blood to the head had been cut off for at least a minute or so. Lisa had been a hair's breadth from death. The risk that a child's heart will stop beating due to lack of oxygen is greater than with an adult. Injuries were also found in the genital area.

BEING ARRESTED

When Eckard was arrested he denied the accusations, despite the overwhelming evidence against him. Lisa identified him in a line-up. A pill box of an unusual brand was found on the scene of the crime. It was the same brand of pills that Eckard always took for his acid stomach. There was also a rough draft of an anonymous letter in Eckard's home, a confused letter which he sent to the police after the crime.

Even the least violent offenders – flashers, peeping Toms and those who abuse children verbally – are compensating for the abuse they themselves have been subjected to. This compulsive staging of an inner fantasy of being important, powerful and dangerous drives the perpetrator to go farther and take greater risks.

Paradoxically enough, the offender may have an unconscious yearning to be apprehended by the police. The violated penis looks big and mighty in the blue glow of a police car's flashing lights. Eckard came close to murdering a little girl. He left a clear trail of evidence behind.

He was stopped, at least temporarily, from further escalating a compulsive behaviour whose ultimate consequences he came close to realizing and which even perhaps frightened him.

9. Central areas and themes of therapy

At the Boys' Clinic we have set aside a separate room which allows the visiting boys to give free vent to their inner lives in a safe environment. A room that allows free reign for the imagination and stimulates open-hearted discussion, movement, emotional expression and reflection.

The boys we work with often have a need for strongly aggressive expressions in play and movement. This means that things can sometimes get pretty wild.

The children's trust in adults has been damaged. It can take time to build it up again. Both the children and their parents may harbour suspicions towards men.

It happens that children are worried because they aren't sure whether we might try to do "dirty stuff" with them when they are left alone with us in the therapy room. The situation where a mother turns her boy over to the therapist bears a certain resemblance to the situation where the same mother turned the same boy over to the man who then abused him. We must mention this analogy in order to overcome any suspicions that may exist. Even though the worry and suspicion are not clearly expressed, conversations with the children and parents indicate that these fears are often present.

Since most of the boys we meet have been exploited by men, this threshold must to be crossed in order to establish a trusting therapeutic relationship.

But once this is achieved, we believe it is an advantage in these contexts to be a male therapist, in view of the possibilities for alternative male identification.

STEPPING-STONES

We have found in our treatment work at the Boys' Clinic that there are certain central areas and themes of therapy that serve as crucial stepping-stones in the therapeutic journey. They can be summed-up by the following four points:

- Describing the abuse

- Expressing feelings

- Saying no and setting boundaries

- Acceptance

We have sorted the therapeutic themes we encounter in our work and use as stepping-stones under these four headings. These themes are not sharply delineated from each other. In many cases they can be said to constitute different aspects of the same problem.

Themes such as these are common to all therapeutic work. Some of them may be more specific for children/boys who have been subjected to sexual abuse.

The stepping-stone model is meant to be understood as depicting different dimensions of the therapy, processes that have different focuses and can lead into each other sequentially, recur or run concurrently. It expresses how the treatment process can be divided into "areas".

Some schools of therapy advocate a detached, non-controlling posture on the part of the therapist. But our experience is that with these boys there is so much resistance, denial and aversion to approaching therapeutically relevant material that an excessively detached posture does nothing to move the process forward. The therapy then risks bogging down in an endless series of ping-pong games.

It therefore helps to identify themes such as these, which we can use in a more active and controlling way without necessarily getting stuck in the type of pre-planned "programme" which has to be gone through point-by-point or step-by-step and which, despite its therapeutic effects, can sometimes be experienced as mechanical or stereotyped.

DESCRIBING THE ABUSE

Describing the abuse is a way of "making reality real". Here the children make use of various means of expression, depending on age and disposition. For some boys, language is the best way, describing in words the abusive acts to which they have been subjected. Others prefer to show in play what they have experienced, especially the younger children who have not yet started school. For yet others, the best means of expression is drawing or using dolls to show what happened. We have anatomically correct dolls and plenty of drawing paper, crayons and pens. The boys can sit at the table or spread out paper and lie on the floor and draw.

Some boys may find it next to impossible to describe the abuse by any means.

Secrets

It is then that secrets become an important therapeutic theme. One of the biggest obstacles in getting children to describe what they have been through is the fact that the abuse has often been shrouded in secrecy and associated with shame and various threats of retribution if they tell. Getting into a discussion of good and bad secrets may help the children.

Good and healthy secrets are exciting to have: The location of a clubhouse, what your little brother is getting for his birthday, etc.

Bad, unhealthy secrets can give you nightmares and make you scared and worried. Children shouldn't have to keep bad secrets. They should be told to an adult, even if you've promised to keep quiet. Otherwise they'll be hard to forget and the fear won't go away.

But the children may not just feel shame and/or guilt, they may simply have decided that this is nothing to talk about. In that case we don't try to push them to talk about something they neither want to nor can bear to talk about. Instead we can show them what we already know and what they've already said by referring to records of police interrogations or other investigation materials, and then sit back and wait for them to come around.

Forgetting

How inclined boys are to tell what happened varies in different periods during the therapy. In the beginning of the treatment process they may describe the abuse, only to "forget" later on and be reluctant to approach the subject. Then at the end of the therapy they may be able to describe what has happened, but now often with details that were not included before.

Describing the abuse is therefore something that should be returned to throughout the treatment process. When sexual abuse is "forgotten", it has a tendency to be transformed into clinical symptoms instead.

Dissociation

Dissociation is another treatment theme in this context. It is associated with the actual telling and description of the abuse. The process of telling activates the coping mechanisms of detachment and splitting-off which the child has used on the abuse occasions (see Chapter 10).

EXPRESSING FEELINGS

We devote a great deal of effort to helping the children to express and describe the feelings associated with the abuse. This is of course one of the cornerstones of all therapy.

We have a wide variety of materials to help the children express their feelings, such as boxing gloves, swords and clubs to hit mattresses with, to help them act out feelings of anger. This coincides to a large extent with Harvey's (1990) recommendations for dynamic play therapy.

We have carefully selected small stuffed animals which the smaller children can use when playing and telling stories as symbols of good and evil, danger and safety, fear and courage, trust and distrust. We also have large stuffed animals, a family of life-sized bears, a life-sized Saint Bernard dog, and a snake as large as a boa constrictor. Besides acting as symbols, the big animals are more physically challenging than the small ones.

The rooms are also equipped with transparent pieces of fabric of various colours that can be used to visualize feelings. Fear can be red and anger white, and when fear turns into anger it is easy to change to a different bit of fabric.

We have pillows, cushions and folding mattresses that can be used to build forts. A five-metre long rubber hose encased in fabric can be used as a rope or a lasso to pull on from two directions to show how it feels when two wills are at war with each other.

In our parachute, a real one of genuine balloon satin, the children can swing, wind down and land, both physically and emotionally.

We collect pictures that express different feelings we can talk about. We have cards with incomplete sentences; pick a card and tell about something that makes you glad, sad, mad, scared, etc. Books of fairy-tales are of course also useful in capturing feelings.

A variety of therapeutic themes can come up during the work of expressing emotions.

Guilt and complicity

In our eagerness to relieve the child of guilt, there may be a risk that we disregard the child's own feeling of complicity in the abuse, which should not be confused with the fact that the abuser is absolutely and fully to blame for what has happened. If it so happens that it was the child who sought out the abuser and perhaps even took the initiative, this is also a part of reality. It can be made comprehensible to the child and must be separated from the questions of responsibility, blame and guilt (see Chapter 17).

Shame, self-image, feelings of being different and worse

All abuse has not necessarily been associated with terror, fear and pain. We meet many boys who have been subjected to "fondling" abuse, which has led them to feel complicit in the crime and worse than their friends and given them a self-image that is tinged with disgust, aversion and confusion (see Chapters 4, 14 and 15).

Inward- and outward-directed aggression

Boys who have been victims of sexual abuse are not infrequently overcome with aggression and hostility, the urge to fight and destroy. When the aggression is not directed towards the abuser, there is a risk it will be directed into destructive channels.

It can be directed outward towards non-abusive parents, towards friends and adults in the neighbourhood and in school, towards pets or inanimate objects.

The anger can be directed inward in the form of various degrees of self-destructiveness. The boy may be involved in an inordinate number of accidents, he may deliberately injure himself, and sometimes the self-destructive actions may lead to attempted or successful suicide.

Sexual acting-out

Many boys who have been referred to us as victims of sexual abuse have also turned out to be abusers themselves. And conversely, boys who have been remitted to us as young offenders have sometimes been found to have been victims themselves. Investigating and trying to understand the often very short path from victim to perpetrator is an inescapable theme of therapy (see Chapters 3, 12 and 25).

Abuser's two faces

Exploring the child's feelings towards the abuser often entails splitting the father into two persons: One is a good daddy who could sometimes be an "ordinary" daddy whom the child could love and can still miss sometimes, and the other is a bad daddy whom the child is afraid of and furious with for what he has done (see Chapter 16).

Fear

Sexually abused children are often frightened children. Their fears can vary in degree and root cause.

Some children may be afraid that the perpetrator will seek retribution for the fact that they have told.

Some children may be afraid of being abandoned.

Some children may be afraid of getting in touch with the fear they felt when they were being sexually abused.

Some children may be afraid of nightmares or vague catastrophes (see Chapters 3, 11, 16 and 20).

HOMOSEXUALITY

For a boy, being subjected to sexual abuse by a man or a boy can often lead to reflections about homosexuality. Is it "catching"? Why did he choose me? Do I look like a queer? and so on. Sometimes such questions can crop up several years after the abuse when the boy is approaching adolescence and is beginning to comprehend what happened to him in a different way (see Chapters 17 and 18).

Fight, flight, protection

Fight, flight and protection are themes that come up in conjunction with the treatment of traumatized children who have been subjected to painful and frightening sexual assaults where they have been prevented from fighting, fleeing or protecting themselves during the assault (see Chapters 11 and 13).

SAYING NO AND SETTING BOUNDARIES

One thing common to all the boys who visit us is that they have been invaded physically and/or emotionally in one way or another. Anyone who has had his spatial, somatic and emotional territory violated in this manner is at risk himself of violating other people's boundaries. They need help in identifying and expressing emotions that have to do with wanting and not wanting, saying yes and saying no, putting oneself in other people's shoes, private areas and boundaries on the body and in life. Boundaries are an important theme in this treatment area.

We mark boundaries in the room with the big rubber band. We can create areas, "countries", for different emotions and activities which we can move between, explore and play around. We have also learned that many of these boys lack knowledge about their own body and its functions. We sometimes get questions concerning elementary sexual knowledge: "What's the white slimy cream that comes out of my big brother's penis?" or "Why do penises get straight?"

It is our opinion that the treatment must also include pedagogical elements. For this purpose we have books about the human body and certain other publications to serve as a basis for discussion and instruction.

Finally, these children must also learn to get on with their lives, to avoid getting bogged down in victim identity, to reconcile themselves to what has happened and put it behind them, to give up the idea that the past can be remade or denied and to accept the fact that complete justice can never be obtained.

It is not at all certain that sexually abused children will ever be able to accept and become reconciled to their fate. Many will probably carry their rage, their fear and above all their shame within them for a long time to come.

The idea of acceptance and reconciliation is an expression of our belief in a possible way out of powerlessness. Here the boys need a great deal of support from those around them to be able to accept themselves as normal, ordinary boys, in spite of the unusual and abnormal experiences they have been through (see Chapter 20). It is important that sexually molested boys also be able to do the things that all other boys do: swim, bicycle or play football. They also have to learn how to tell time and to tie their own shoes.

There is a risk that not only the boy, but also those around him, will get stuck in the idea that the abuse is the cause of all their problems. The abuse is taken as an excuse for an incapacitating overprotection without reasonable expectations and demands. All foolish and age-inadequate behaviour is excused by the abuse.

Acceptance and reconciliation are just as difficult and necessary for all the helping adults in the abused child's life. We try to make this process clear by also doing normal, ordinary things at the Boys' Clinic. We have milk and cookies and talk about hobbies and future plans, just to underscore the fact that even if you've been subjected to abnormal, disgusting things and been referred to us for that reason, you don't have to be abnormal or disgusting yourself.

An important part of acceptance is allowing oneself to grieve over the fact that everything ought to have been different. Longing for a father or grief at never having had one is a universal theme in the therapy at the Boys' Clinic.

64

Boys who have been abused by their biological father long for a "nice" father. Boys who have been abused by their mother long for a normal mother and wish there had been a father there who had understood and been able to intervene on their behalf. Grief and longing become important themes in this area of treatment, and naturally also the hope that, despite the abnormal nature of what has happened, it will be possible to live a good life and feel like a normal boy.

Rituals
Rituals can help people to accept and put their problems behind them. Letting a child say good-bye to the abuser in the therapy room can be one way. Often the children pick one of the big teddy-bears to be the abuser. The selected "abuser bear" then becomes the object of a great deal of aggression and other emotions. At a certain point in the therapy it may also be time to say good-bye to the abuser, to take the teddy-bear out of the therapy room and turn to other matters. When the teddy-bear is carried out, feelings of grief and loss may come to the surface.

Our clinic is situated on the top floor of a tall building. Some of the windows cannot be opened for safety reasons. But at the end of a therapy session we sometimes make a little paper swallow which we symbolically burden with all the fears and emotions associated with the abuse. We open one of those windows that are not supposed to be opened and we launch the little paper swallow so that it is borne away forever on the winds of the world...

10. Making reality real

This is a transcript from a police interrogation with Henry, seven years old. He had been the victim of very severe abuse by Larry, the father in the foster home where he was placed.

Police: How did it begin?
Henry: Larry got into my bed, even though I didn't want him to.
P: What happened then?
H: He told me to sit on his willy.
P: What happened then?
H: That's what I don't dare tell.
P: How does it feel when you think about this?
H: It feels strange.
P: How?
H: When I turn it feels as if I am walking straight ahead.
P: Did he say anything to you?
H: He said to stick my willy in his behind. That was what I thought hurt. When he tried to pull down the skin.
P: Did he have any Vaseline?
H: Yes.
P: What did he do with the Vaseline?
H: He smeared it into his own behind.
P: And what happened then?
H: He told me to pull in and out on his willy.
P: What happened after Larry had smeared in the Vaseline?

H: He told me to stick my willy in there.

P: Did you do it?

H: Yes, otherwise he said he would hit me.

P: How was your willy when you stuck it in?

H: It was down.

P: Was it hard or soft?

H: It was soft.

P: Did anything else happen?

H: No, I don't remember anything.

P: Did you smell anything special?

H: When I had to put my arm in his behind it smelled like poop on my hand.

P: How much of your hand went into his behind?

H: About up to here (shows elbow and then hides arm and hand inside jumper).

P: Did anything else happen?

H: That's stuff I don't remember.

P: Did you have to hold his willy other times?

H: It was on Tvärgatan when he was sitting in a swivel chair.

P: What happened then?

H: I had to hold it and do like this (shows masturbating motions with arm). Some white stuff came out.

P: Where did it come out?

H: Out of the top.

P: The top of what.

H: His willy, the top of his willy.

P: Did Larry ever put his willy anywhere else?

H: (thinks) In my mouth too. He wanted my willy in his mouth.

P: Tell me how it happened.

H: He said I should pee. Only a little came out.

P: Where were you supposed to pee?

H: Into his mouth.

P: Do you remember how your willy was then?

H: It was up then.

P: Where was Larry then?

68

H: He sat on the toilet lid, but he had lifted up the cover.

P: How was Larry's willy then?

H: It was standing up.

P: What happened then?

H: He said I should sit on his willy. Then when I sat down, I said: "Ow, I don't want to."

P: Did Larry say anything then?

H: He said "Quiet!" And a bad word: "Shut up!" That was when he lifted me up like this and licked my behind and said I should lick his willy.

P: And what happened then?

H: I got a stomach-ache because it tasted icky. I felt like I was going to throw up then.

P: Did you say anything to Larry then?

H: I said I wanted to get bigger.

P: Did Larry tell you not to say anything about this?

H: He said if I told he would kill himself.

RECOGNIZING REALITY

This conversation has to do with the details of what Henry has been through, how it felt, how it smelled, what it sounded like, what it looked like.

What Larry did with Henry had been Henry's secret. Larry had threatened to kill himself if Henry told. So he kept quiet. If Larry hadn't gone to the police himself and confessed, his abuse of Henry might never have been revealed. Telling wasn't an option for Henry. His only option was to try to turn the abusive episodes into non-events, something that hadn't happened. The consequence of these attempts at suppression were symptoms such as nightmares, difficulties concentrating, self-destructiveness and detachment.

His schoolwork was suffering, he was constantly having accidents, falling out of trees or off roofs, cutting himself with knives. Everyone around him could see he was a troubled child, but they couldn't see he was a victim of sexual abuse.

Does a police interrogation, where all the details of the abuse have to be described by the child in his own words, have any therapeutic value? We think it does. The police interrogation helps the child make reality real. It counteracts the dissociative defences which the child used to protect his psyche when the abuse occurred, but which become a handicap in daily life.

Dissociating is a very fundamental and effective defence against an intolerable reality. The dissociative reactions are activated and become the victim's protection on the actual occasions of abuse. Separating the emotions from the event is one way to cope and survive.

Anyone who has been with a very small child at a hospital during a painful examination knows that when the child realizes that screaming doesn't help it may suddenly fall asleep instead.

Adults sometimes describe how, during abuse or torture, they have experienced the sensation of leaving their body, gone into a trance or seen themselves from the outside so that the assaults have "only" afflicted the body and not the inner person. "Tunnel vision" or "spacing out" are other dissociative phenomena described by Hunter (1990).

NON-EVENTS

Furniss (1991) has experienced that children often describe how the abuse took place in total silence, without eye contact, in the dark and with stereotyped repetitions and rituals. This is a means of turning the abuse into a non-event and denying it or splitting it off so that the child is not in touch with any emotions surrounding the abuse. The contrast between the intense physical sensations during the abuse I pain, sexual arousal, anxiety and fear due to an ability to leave the scene I and the total silence and lack of contact between victim and abuser contribute towards splitting off the abuse from reality.

By minimizing all other impressions, the abuser negates the reality of the ongoing abuse. "What is going on now is not really happening at all." The child may experience that the abuser suddenly becomes a different person just before committing the sexual act. Voice, gestures and facial expressions suddenly change from something familiar to something strange and frightening. By splitting off the abusive acts from reality by becoming "the other person", by psychologically shielding the child, the abuser denies the child the opportunity to perceive reality as reality and to name the abuse as abuse.

We at the Boys' Clinic have benefitted a great deal from the records of good police interrogations. When the police have made reality real in documented interrogations, we as therapists can use the material to keep a grip on what really happened in the therapy work, which largely has to do with integrating and processing emotions. The police interrogation thereby becomes the first therapeutic counterattack against the strong internal and external forces striving to sweep the abusive events under the carpet at the price of a disoriented and dissociated patient.

IS IT TRUE OR AM I MAKING IT UP?

"The worst of it is that sometimes I don't know whether I'm telling the truth or making things up. Sometimes it feels as if I've dreamt everything," said Henry at the Boys' Clinic. In this case the perpetrator had at least confessed, but if he hadn't, Henry's statement could have diminished his legal credibility. For us it was an indication of a dissociative defence. When he said that he didn't know if it was true or not, he showed us how he had managed to stand Larry's abuse for such a long time. He had developed the ability to sometimes erase the sexual acts from his memory.

PHYSICAL SYMPTOMS

Clear physical symptoms can sometimes also be a manifestation of dissociative reactions. For example, it may sometimes feel as if certain parts of the body start to grow, get warm, tickle or no longer belong to the body. "When I turn it feels as if I am walking straight ahead," said Henry. Henry felt as if his body split in two and the halves walked in different directions. Other sexually exploited children have expressed the same feeling like this: "It feels as if my arms didn't belong to my body" or "my hands feel enormous, bigger than the rest of my body".

Children can talk about very severe abuse and traumatic events completely without emotion. Such a manner of speaking can be interpreted as indicating either that the child has made up what is being said, or that the child has been told to memorize what to say by someone else. In either case what the child says lacks credibility.

We believe that it may just as well be exactly the opposite, that such a "mechanical way of telling" may be an expression of dissociation from an intolerable reality. The child puts itself in a similar dissociative state during the abusive events. The appropriate feelings would be far too intolerable for the child to harbour and express when the abuse is mentioned.

11. The phoney policeman

In the introductory chapter "The phoney policeman", we talked about Patrik, who was sexually abused by a stranger in the doorway of the block of flats where he lived. The symptoms Patrik suffered after the abuse were:

- Extreme fear, manifested in nightmares, fear of strange men, fear of sleeping in his own bed, fear that the perpetrator was hiding in the flat, and fear that he would seek revenge.
- Troublesome olfactory sensations. He perceived that strange men had the same odour as the perpetrator had. When he recognized the smell he got scared. After the abuse, Patrik compulsively smelled things he touched.
- Blinking tic. At the time of the assault, Patrik had shut his eyes tightly and turned his head aside.

FEAR GOT THE UPPER HAND

Patrik was a traumatized child. The feeling of terror he had experienced during the abuse had burnt itself into his mind. He couldn't get rid of his fear. Even though he knew the perpetrator was in prison, he was still afraid he was standing behind the shower curtain or hiding under his bed.

"I know it isn't so, it just feels like it," said Patrik. His fear was stronger than his reason.

The therapist suggested that Patrik should keep the kitchen knives

73

next to his bed until he felt certain that the perpetrator would not come back for revenge.

At Patrik's second visit the blinking tic had become worse. Three weeks had now passed since the assault. He had started hitting his eyes hard with his finger. He hit until it hurt. Patrik thought the eyelid had begun to "hang" more than before. The number of strange men he was afraid of had increased. More men he had come near had smelled just like the perpetrator.

His fear had increased. He now slept every night in his mother's bed. He kept the knives next to his own bed.

SLASHED WILDLY AT THE TEDDY-BEAR

In the playroom at the Boys' Clinic, Patrik built a replica of his bedroom. A mattress represented his bed, and the red and white parachute was his cover. The big brown teddy-bear became the perpetrator who came in through the window. Patrik attacked the teddy-bear with a sword. He slashed wildly at the teddy-bear. The therapist encouraged Patrik to say what he felt when he was hitting the teddy-bear.

"You slimeball! You aren't going to do that anymore. You pig! Go home and fuck your girlfriend instead. No, I take it back, you don't have a girlfriend! You shouldn't mess around with kids!"

"Slimeball! Pig!"

Patrik slashed at the teddy-bear where his genitals would have been if he had had any. He slashed and shrieked.

Then Patrik made a drawing of the abusive act. A frightened boy who looks glad. The boy masturbates the perpetrator. "Shake" [English word wrote Patrik on the picture. Asked what "shake" meant he answered that it meant "jerk off", but he thought it was too nasty to write it in Swedish.

When he had drawn the incident, he was asked to draw how the little boy in the picture could escape or defeat the perpetrator. Patrik then drew a boy with a spray can in his hand with "knockout drops" that he sprays on the perpetrator. The perpetrator puts his hands over his eyes and falls down. When the perpetrator is lying on the ground, the boy sticks a sword in his stomach. The perpetrator is shown bleeding, "blood and fat" runs out of his stomach.

Patrik's imagination now got carried away. The perpetrator was dead, but that wasn't enough. He was to be thrown into a rubbish container and sent to Africa. There his body was to be strung on a big hook and thrown into the ocean to the sharks. When the sharks had eaten up his body, his skeleton was to be put in another box.

"And then what happens?" asked the therapist.

"Then he comes alive again," replied Patrik.

OLD FEARS

Patrik wasn't able to kill his fear that easily. Patrik killed the perpetrator over and over again in the therapy room, but he always came back to life. There was no improvement in Patrik's state of anxiety during the first few months. The tic, the fear of strangers and the olfactory sensations persisted. What kind of internal processes had the abuse set in motion? Was there anything in Patrik's earlier history that could explain why we weren't able to cure his symptoms?

Patrik had two older brothers. His father travelled a great deal. Perhaps Patrik had tried to be older than he was? Perhaps like many other boys with older brothers he had suppressed fears normal for his age so that he could measure up to and compete with his older brothers, especially the one who was only a year and a half older? Patrik had always been an unusually self-assured and bold little boy. Now the abuse triggered both old, suppressed fears and new fears. The incident gave Patrik a legitimate excuse to be frightened and timid. He was allowed to be in the centre of the family and the one who needed help.

The therapist suggested to his mother that Patrik should be treated for a while as a slightly younger child than his ten years. He should be given more motherly care and be pampered and coddled more by everyone in the family. But he should also be given more rules to obey. He should have to go to bed earlier, be at home more and so on. Just as if he were a few years younger. Patrik became "smaller" for a couple of months. Then he got tired of the game and wanted to be ten years old again.

After six months the eye tic faded away. The knives found their way back to the kitchen drawer where they belonged. Patrik slept sometimes in his own bed, sometimes in his mother's. His fear of strangers abated, but did not go away completely. The olfactory sensations took the longest time to abate.

After eight months, the therapy was terminated on Patrik's own initiative. He was promised that he could come back if he changed his mind. When he concluded therapy, Patrik had a habit of reflexively smelling everything he touched – pens, cutlery, etc.

At that point in time, the perpetrator had served his sentence and was out of prison. Patrik's fear was more appropriate now. He was afraid of meeting the perpetrator, but he was no longer afraid that the perpetrator would come in through the window at night.

James (1989) emphasizes the importance of offering traumatized children treatment over a long period of time, though not continuously.

A child will respond to a traumatic event in different ways depending on its age. It is not possible to bring about a therapeutic resolution of problems that have not yet surfaced.

In Patrik's case, the therapeutic objective was that he should overcome some of his fear, including the more annoying symptoms, that he should learn to evaluate risk situations in a reasonably realistic fashion and that he should be given an opportunity to find an outlet for emotions that were related to the abuse.

What happened with the perpetrator? He was a recidivist. He had been convicted of sexual offences against children six times. Sometimes he had been sentenced to short prison terms, sometimes to care. This time he received a seven-month prison sentence.

12. Trauma and compulsory repetition

Carl was seven years old. His sister was ten. His sister was reading aloud from one of the evening tabloids about a murder case – a fratricide. A girl had been strangled by her brother when he came home from school. Carl was very upset by the story. He imagined himself in the girl's situation and said:

"You come home from school, all happy, and you wonder what you're going to have for dinner, and then you get strangled!"

When he said it he got more upset. He grabbed a pencil and a piece of paper and quickly made a drawing where his little sister comes in through the door with her schoolbag, takes a couple of steps, is assaulted and then strangled. He was very concentrated as he drew, and when he was finished he gave the drawing to his father. Then he went out to play.

We think that this example illustrates a successful attempt to deal with a very small trauma, the type of "everyday trauma" to which children are frequently exposed and which they have the resources to handle.

When his sister read the story of the murder aloud to him, Carl identified with the murdered girl and became frightened. He both talked about and made a drawing of the frightening event. He gave the drawing to his father, who thereby "saw" and became the receptacle of his son's fear. Then Carl was able to leave the event and go on.

THE CONCEPT OF TRAUMA
The world "trauma" comes from the Greek word for "wound" and can mean either a physical injury (wound) to living tissue caused by an

external agent or a psychological injury stemming from a frightening experience.

James (1989) defines trauma as an overwhelming, uncontrollable experience which affects the victim psychologically by inducing feelings of helplessness, vulnerability, loss of safety and loss of control.

Intense fear and/or intense physical pain, in combination with powerlessness, are the main ingredients of a traumatic experience in the psychological sense.

Examples of traumatic events may be war or, the sudden death of a loved one, separations or frightening near-death experiences. Children may also be traumatized by situations which adults may not experience as particularly frightening, for example getting accidentally separated from their mothers at a department store or being frightened by an older brother or sister. Stories about war or murder on television or in the newspaper may also trigger traumatic experiences, such as in the example with Carl.

FOUR FACTORS

Not everyone is traumatized by the same events. Cullberg (1975) points out four factors that are of importance in a traumatic crisis situation:

1. The triggering situation
2. The inner, private significance of the occurrence for the traumatized individual, interwoven with his or her life history.
3. The particular point in his or her life or development in which the individual finds himself.
4. The social circumstances and associated family situation of the traumatized individual.

Typical symptoms that can be traced to traumatic events constitute what is known as "post-traumatic stress syndrome", PTSD. These symptoms are nightmares, inability to concentrate, motoric restlessness, panic reactions, various states of somatic pain and tension, and flashbacks, where clear pictures of the frightening event are replayed almost like a film loop in the mind.

78

COMPULSIVE REPETITION

Mangs and Martell (1990) describe compulsive repetition, which is a type of obsessive-compulsive reaction. Psychologically, compulsive repetition is dynamically linked to a trauma. The compulsion is driven by suppressed impulses from traumatic situations which strive over and over again to overcome the trauma and achieve resolution of the unresolved. The compulsion obtains its strength from unresolved frightening experiences where the individual and those near him have failed to deal with the anxiety created by the frightening event. The anxiety lives on and is temporarily abated in repetition rituals based on the same theme as the original trauma. For the traumatized individual, overcoming his anxiety may be a lifelong task.

The repetition situations arise when the traumatized person encounters situations similar to the original, traumatic one, or when the person seeks out and stages events that resemble those that have caused the fear and anxiety. At best, compulsive repetition is a healing process where the effects of the trauma are gradually incorporated into the individual's personality.

At worst, the compulsion is a destructive force that only temporarily relieves the anxiety. It is a force that drives the individual into a destructive repetitious behaviour based on the same theme as the original trauma.

One of the adult men who have contacted us told how he had been subjected to anal rape at the age of thirteen.

Now thirty years old, he was still driven by a compulsion to drive in his car to the site of the rape. He was then overwhelmed by the same feelings as when it happened, that he was dying and had intensive pains around his anus. Sometimes he would get an urge to let go of the steering wheel and relinquish control of the car. By returning to the scene of the traumatic experience, he was trying over and over again to find a solution to the desperate powerlessness he still carried within him.

RICHARD AND THE DOLL

Another example is Richard, five years old, who was sexually molested by Lars, a male childminder at the day nursery. The childminder locked himself in the nap room with Richard. There he pulled down Richard's trousers and abused him anally. This had apparently happened several times before he was caught in the act by a woman colleague.

Back home Richard had a doll. Almost every day Richard wanted to be left alone in his room with the doll.

"Now I want to be alone and think about Lars," said Richard. In such situations his parents were not allowed to enter the room; if they did he would get angry. His parents were curious and peeked through the keyhole. There they saw their five-year-old son undress the doll, take out his penis and press it against the doll's bottom.

Compulsive repetition as a healing force can become problematic when the child has been subjected to sexual abuse, which is by its nature secret. Repeating secrets, as Richard did when he locked himself in with the doll, is not reparative if the repetition has to be done in secret. The child is then not "seen" when it tries to deal with its fear. It does not have an opportunity to "hand over" its fear to a secure and strong parent, as Carl did.

Nor, in Richard's case, is it a question of play that alleviates anxiety, but rather an attempt at anxiety alleviation where the secrecy and solitude of the repetition ritual instead heightens the individual's anxiety. His secrecy indicates fear of being punished for his actions. He doesn't get rid of his fear, but continues repeating the same destructive attempts at resolution, which aggravate rather than repair the injuries he has suffered from the abuse.

Some sexually abused boys that have come to the Boys' Clinic have in turn abused younger children during or after the period they were being abused. The compulsive repetition can allow the sexually abused boy to play the role of abuser. By subjecting others to what he himself has suffered, he blocks his own feeling of vulnerability and fear. This impairs his chances of dealing with his own trauma productively.

DENIED EMOTIONS

As we see, denied fears and denied feelings of vulnerability are the greatest obstacles to dealing productively with traumatic events. In the mind of a child, things that can't be expressed in words often don't exist, and the best way to forget a frightening event is to not talk about it. The child may get frightened all over again if we talk about it. But in the silence of denied emotions surrounding traumatic events, we believe the risk is greater that the victim will get stuck in destructive repetitions.

13. The struggle against El Loco

Marcus was four years old, his family came from Uruguay and they had applied for asylum in Sweden. They lived in a refugee compound. One day, Marcus accompanied his father to the course in Swedish that was being held at a school not far from the compound. He had done so before and he was not unfamiliar with the surroundings. After a while Marcus left the classroom. His father wasn't worried; there wasn't any harm in the boy's playing for a while in the corridor.

But Marcus when off on his own and ran into a teenage boy who was a total stranger to him. The boy lured Marcus into a shower room where he took off his trousers and forced the boy to submit to anal intercourse.

The father found his son with his trousers down crying in the shower room. At first, Marcus couldn't explain what had happened, but when his mother came he told. The event was reported to the police and the perpetrator was identified and arrested.

AFRAID OF EVERYTHING

When the family came to the Boys' Clinic, the parents said that after the abuse Marcus had become afraid of "everything". He was afraid to be alone, he couldn't do things he had done before and he hid behind his parents every time he saw a strange man. He was restless, had difficulty sleeping, had nightmares and had uncontrolled fits of rage directed at both his mother and his father, and he didn't dare assert himself against other children.

In the playroom at the Boys' Clinic, Marcus played distractedly with

83

whatever he came across. He turned boxes upside down, pulled things off shelves and wanted to run out of the room. His parents were very insecure and didn't know how to deal with Marcus after what had happened. They thought that everything he did was due to the harmful effects of the rape and they were afraid to cause him any further distress by setting limits for him. They were worried about what would happen with him in the future, what harmful after-effects he might have.

SETTING LIMITS

The therapist urged the parents to set limits for Marcus, make demands on him, but to be careful to listen to what he had to say; not to blame him for going with someone he didn't know, and to allow him to be angry but not to injure himself or anyone else.

The parents also wondered why the boy had become so changed and aggressive. The therapist answered that four-year-olds don't realize that their parents aren't omniscient. Marcus might believe that his parents knew what was happening and let it happen, and for that he was now furious with them.

Marcus's symptoms were fear, inability to concentrate and nightmares. He was afraid of everything and wanted more than anything to hide on his mother's lap. The therapeutic task was to make a cautious attempt to approach the traumatic event again.

The following two sessions were devoted to establishing a trusting relationship with Marcus, getting to know him. Marcus thought it was fun to play fantasy and role games, which indicated that he had the resources to process what he had been through. He still didn't want to talk about what had happened, didn't want to demonstrate with dolls, draw or describe the abusive act in any other way. The therapist asked if he knew what kind of a place the Boys' Clinic was. He didn't. His parents had said that they were going to visit friends, where he would be able to play.

The therapist then urged the parents to tell Marcus that this is a place where boys come who have had something terrible done to them by a bigger person, something that has hurt and frightened them. And when the therapist plays with the children, it's because he knows it's a good way for the children not to feel so afraid and worried as many children do who have been through something terrible.

When his mother told this to Marcus he sat on her lap, looked down, grew completely quiet and looked sad. When the therapist asked if he wanted to come back and play now that he knew what kind of place it was, he didn't reply at first. Then he whispered:

"I do, but not for so long."

When Marcus had been told "what kind of a place this was", it proved to have a dramatic effect on the content and intensity of his games. It was as if he understood what the time could be used for, and that gave him some kind of hope.

From the case notes after the fourth visit:

Marcus is beginning to play with the stuffed animals and deciding which ones are to be his friends and then the shark and the crocodile | "cocodrile" | have to be enemies and attack the nice animals. It is Marcus who rules over the nice animals. They are very strong and always win over the "cocodrile" and the shark. Good struggles against evil and wins because good is much stronger.

Then the game changes. This struggle is between Marcus and me. He wants me to try to capture him with the red ribbon. He seems to enjoy this cat-and-mouse game immensely. He shrieks and laughs. He is on the whole much tougher, more open and unafraid than when he first came here, silent, timid and hardly daring do anything.

THE PERPETRATOR IS GIVEN A NAME

A breakthrough was made at the next session. Marcus and his parents had given a name to his abuser: El Loco, the crazy one.

After having told this to the therapist, Marcus starting using the name in his games, which evolved into increasingly violent showdowns and executions of El Loco during ensuing visits. Sometimes Marcus himself played the part of El Loco.

On some occasions he didn't want to fight the crazy one at all, preferring to play tabletop ice hockey with the therapist instead. Then the therapist might do no more than ask if the big brown teddy-bear could watch, and Marcus would take up the struggle against El Loco again.

One time, when he was occupied most intensively with trying to kill the crazy one in various ways, Marcus suddenly sought eye contact with the therapist and pressed a toy rifle into the teddy-bear's bottom and fired a shot. This was his way of telling the therapist what the crazy one had done to him. The therapist asked:

"Was that what it felt like when the crazy one was bad to you?"

Marcus nodded silently and the therapist and Marcus were eventually able to express in words what had happened.

PARENTS HELP

Now that Marcus and the therapist had words for what had happened to him the treatment could enter a new phase. He had received assistance in making reality real for him. Now it was important for him to keep his grip on this reality and then explore ways of getting help with all his other problems, such as his temper tantrums, his fear, etc. Here it was important to enlist the aid of his parents.

During the sixth and seventh sessions, Marcus continued playing games based on the theme "The struggle against El Loco", except that now his mother and father got to take part, by turns as the victim and as El Loco, or by coming to Marcus's aid when he needed it in the struggle. Now the games were based on the theme of protection and control.

Marcus enjoyed being in total control of the events during the game and moving freely between being the victim and being the attacker, between fighting alone and accepting help. In conversations afterward, the parents could then assure Marcus that they would protect him from other madmen, that no one would be able to hurt him anymore.

From the case notes after the eighth visit:

*Marcus is still afraid of strangers, hides behind his mother and father.
Furthermore he is aggressive towards his parents. He wants to fight
the crazy one today, dress up in armour and attack from inside the
house he has built, then he wants to tie up the crazy one with a piece of
string he has brought with him. Then he ties me up. Then we start
talking about what the crazy one has done with him, he shows me and*

86

*we talk about the words for willy and bottom in Spanish. Then he
wants to fight. First carefully with me, then violently with his father.
He knees his father in the crotch and kicks him as hard as he can with
his boots. The father gets tears in his eyes and looks distressed and
doesn't know what to do. I urge the father not to let Marcus hurt him
and at the same time urge Marcus to scream at his daddy why he is
angry. "You didn't do anything!" screams Marcus.*

*Once again his father and mother gave Marcus permission to be
just as angry as he was, but they also told him they weren't going to let
him hurt anyone, the way he did to his father just now.*

*Then they played a game where Marcus went into another room
and his parents had to guess what he was doing there. This was to
show him that adults can't know everything that happens just because
they're adults and that's why children have to tell. The session
concluded with Marcus and his father boxing. The father was
instructed to teach Marcus how to fight and what the rules are.*

*Marcus thought this was a lot of fun and didn't want to stop. To
calm himself down he was told to land softly and carefully a few times
in the parachute, and then swing back and forth while his mother and
father held him.*

HE ISN'T IN MY HEAD ANY MORE

The next session was videotaped so that Marcus could see how well he is
able to fight and what a strong daddy and mummy he has who can protect
him. He played as usual with all the animals, staged the battle between
good and evil, executed the crazy one, described in front of the camcorder
what El Loco had done and was then eager to watch the replay of the tape.

When he got to the part where he told about the rape he held his eyes.
When the therapist asked him what it felt like when he held his eyes, he
said that he felt scared, but that El Loco now existed only on the
videotape, since he had been blown up with dynamite.

"He isn't in my head anymore."

At the next visit, the parents said that Marcus was now like a different
boy and that they weren't worried about him anymore. He was calm and
not at all as restless and aggressive as before.

87

As we saw, Marcus himself gave an excellent interpretation of what had happened, the liberating feeling of having exorcised El Loco from his psyche.

On a symbolic plane, he had met El Loco in the playroom and had then had an opportunity to introduce an element that had been missing at the time of the abuse: the means of protecting himself, the ability to struggle and the opportunity to flee. With that he got back his sense of being able to exercise control over his life again. As long as El Loco had free reign inside him, he was deprived of this capability and fixated on the helplessness and horror he had experienced during the abuse. Marcus' struggle against El Loco illustrates how a trauma can be processed and integrated into a painful memory that can be handled; how playing a game can destroy an inner demon.

14. Stigma

— THE SENSE OF BEING DIFFERENT AND INFERIOR

"How could I have been a mother, I who was an orphanage child." This is a woman being interviewed on the radio. She is eighty years old, famous and successful. But the stigma from her childhood in an orphanage had been with her all her life. The shame over not having been loved enough as a small girl had not been expunged, despite a life of social success and recognition. In her own eyes she had never reached the stage of adulthood that daring to become a parent entails. In that respect she branded herself as being different and inferior to other women.

Alexander came to the Boys' Clinic at the age of twelve. His father had abused him sexually for many years. His mother could not have him living with her at home, so he was placed in an institution. Alexander had developed a shamelessness that made him impossible in normal settings. He exposed himself and ran around naked in his neighbourhood, he ran away, urinated and defecated on the floor, and spoke in a partially codified language that only those initiated by him could understand. He had a sexualized behaviour that confused and terrified other children and adults.

RED AND WHITE SHAME

In her book *Rött och Vitt* ("Red and White"), Else-Britt Kjellqvist (1993) analyzes shame and shamelessness.

- "Red shame" is blood-filled and pulsates with life. It helps us to defend our most private and intimate places.

- "White shame" destroys and paralyzes. It is a covenant with death. It penetrates into our most private and intimate places.

"White shame" is the shame of sexual abuse. It is so unbearable that it must be concealed at all costs, distorted and camouflaged beyond recognition so it is safe from insight and renewed violation.

Alexander had been subjected to shameless acts by his father. Now Alexander was himself a shameless child. Why? When Alexander sought his father's love, he got it on one condition I that he submit to his father's sexual lusts. The boy reached out to his father and was accepted only on the condition that he accept his father's shameless acts. His conclusion was that he wasn't worth anything aside from his shamelessness. Being shameless was a defence against the violation he suffered, but also a way of identifying with his father. An opportunity to be someone instead of no one.

Alexander harboured a self-contempt for his own body, his sexuality and his emotions. He denied himself as a human being. This denial was at the core of the personal breakdown which was taking a heavy toll on Alexander himself and those closest to him.

To reach out and get a response is a fundamental need. To offer your love and be rejected as unloved is the worst, the ultimate shame. Kjellqvist describes the connection between shame and pathological narcissism.

The function of shame in narcissistic disturbances is two-fold. Firstly, it provides a driving force for the formation of the grandiose ego, and secondly it is the sense of shame that is responsible for the separation of the grandiose ego from the rest of the personality.

Being unloved, or only being loved on certain terms, is such a painful experience for the child that it must be denied and compensated for. In the feeling of not being loved, the child degrades himself and makes himself inferior. The child assumes guilt for the deficiency in his parents. In compensating, the child splits off his feelings of inferiority, projects them onto others and blows himself up to a shameless, grandiose person.

90

The child makes itself inaccessible to attempts at approach by others, inaccessible to feelings and armoured for defence against new abuse. The price paid by the child for this inaccessibility is a self-dehumanization.

Adam, who had been sexually abused by his mother, now lived in a foster home. He was fifteen years old. He had to shower and wash his hair every morning. It was a compulsion. If he didn't do it he thought he smelled like excrement. This showering had become problematic a couple of months ago. When the water flowed over his head, he felt anxiety. It felt as if someone were trying to drown him. Memory images from his mother's sexualized bathing rituals with him when he was small were mixed with memory images of when she held his head under water.

The memories tormented him so that he couldn't remain under the shower. He wasn't able to soap himself, nor to wash his hair. Nor was he able to refrain from showering, since then he thought he smelled like excrement. His mother had rubbed him with excrement when he was small. Adam coped with the dilemma by walking in and out of the shower with the water turned on. The time during which he stood outside the shower observing the running water grew longer. The process of showering became drawn-out and continued until there was no more hot water. The shower problem created irritation in the foster home. Adam occupied the shower all morning, used up all the hot water and was late for school. Furthermore, he couldn't manage to explain why he had begun showering for such a long time.

Adam was able to shower and wash his hair again when he started to talk about the emotions and memories that came to him in the shower. But his showering remained compulsive. He still thought he smelled like excrement if he didn't shower.

The most basic form of shame is when the child reaches out for its mother and is rejected (Ikonen and Rechardt 1993).

Adam's childhood experience of parental care was one of sexualized interaction with sadistic elements. Adam had not only reached out for his mother and been rejected, he had literally been shat upon.

STIGMA

The word "stigma" comes from Greek and means mark or brand. In ancient Greece, criminals and persons with contagious diseases were branded to mark them as pariahs. The stigmatized were people who were different and inferior to others. We have observed this feeling, which is the hallmark of shame, in almost all the boys that have visited us.

We believe that if a child is sexually abused by a person it loves and is dependent on, that abuse will always be stigmatizing. Instead of meeting the child's needs, the abuser uses the child to satisfy his or her own needs. The child is forced or manipulated into a secret alliance with the abuser. In that alliance the child feels shame, alienation towards what is normal and fear for the consequences of discovery.

The exception to this rule is the relatively few cases where the abuser has been a stranger to the child. Then there has been no relationship of dependence and therefore no emotional betrayal. The child has been tricked or forced into an abusive situation.

For these children, the trauma itself has been the most serious mental injury. The shame has been less pronounced, since the abuse has not been linked to persons near and dear to them. Nor to secrecy.

A LITTLE ABUSE

There are still people today who wonder if a "little" sexual abuse is really so harmful. The kind of abuse, for example, that has been committed by adult paedophiles who have not used violence.

The abuser may be a youth recreation leader, a teacher or a sports coach who takes a great interest in small boys, talks with them, takes them on excursions, invites them home and wins their trust I but then takes advantage of the children's admiration and longing for an adult man who takes an interest in them.

Most paedophilic abuse is not traumatizing in the sense that the children experience great fear or pain in conjunction with the abuse. On the contrary, there are children who feel sexual arousal and experience complicity in the sexual acts. The body can respond sexually to the abuser's fondling. Erection and ejaculation may be the "proof" of the victim's complicity. The external pleasure enhances the internal shame.

92

These children suffer damage that is difficult to repair due to the stigmatizing effect of the abuse.

Children who are forced to repay the youth leader for taking an interest in them with their bodies feel ashamed that they weren't worth loving for their own sake. Furthermore, they are ashamed of their own body's sexual arousal during the abuse. Their self-image is confused and the children seek refuge in wordless compensatory behaviours that are detached from emotions and cause symptoms.

SURRENDERING INDIVIDUALITY

When Olle was seven years old he was assigned to a supportfamily by the social services. His mother was single and had psychological problems. Every other weekend the boy stayed with the support family. Olle liked being there. The father in the support family was kind and took a great interest in Olle, they played computer games and soccer, they built a tree-house.

The first weekend Olle was alone with the support family, the support father came into Olle's bedroom at night, sat down on the edge of the bed, stuck his hand down Olle's pyjama trousers and started fondling his penis.

"He pulled the foreskin back and forth," said Olle when he came to the Boys' Clinic at the age of nine.

This was repeated every time Olle stayed with the support family. The abuse continued for two years before Olle told his mother what was going on. He had always wanted to visit the support family himself. Olle thought the support father was really nice. He had never met his own father. It had been difficult for him to reveal his secret to his mother.

But the secrecy had left its mark in Olle. His self-esteem had suffered, he had complained of headaches and he had begun to lose control of his bowels.

Olle was not sexually demonstrative in his behaviour. He neither shocked nor offended those around him. On the contrary, he was submissive. He was quiet and shy, made an effort to be nice, often went off by himself.

Ikonen and Rechardt note that shame is linked to a desire to hide:

"The innermost essence of shame also harbours the temptation to surrender one's own identity to ensure the esteem of the other person."

93

Olle had surrendered his individuality. He had split off his aggression and parts of his impulsive and spontaneous personality. He shaped his personality in such a way that it would satisfy other people's needs. The support family had been assigned to Olle because Olle's mother was psychologically fragile. Olle could not be demonstrative and shameless. He didn't want to cause worry or be a burden to his already heavily burdened mother. He chose to diminish himself and his needs.

His throbbing headaches and his faecal incontinence can be interpreted as attempts to break out of the inhibiting constraints under which he lived.

15. Kill Larry

How can we come to terms with a self-image that is shameful to talk about?

The therapeutic "antidote" to shame is, as we see it, a long-lasting and dependable therapeutic relationship, where the dependability of the relationship is more important than the content of the therapy. Anton, whom we shall describe in this chapter, experienced every deviation from the routines of his relationship with the Boys' Clinic as a sign of abandonment. A change in the time of his therapy, a forgotten telephone call, a cancellation by the therapist due to an illness in the family led immediately to aggression directed towards others and himself, but not towards the therapist.

"Don't you care about me?" was Anton's constant question, which it took him a long time to dare to ask directly.

Anton was fourteen years old. He had been receiving individual therapy at the Boys' Clinic for three years. He was one of the boys who had been sexually abused from an early age and over a long period of time. He had many problems to struggle with, among them the difference between what was real and what was fantasy. During certain periods when Anton was not feeling well psychologically, fantasy dominated over reality. During such periods, the individual therapy was interrupted and Anton's mother was allowed in the therapy room to help to keep Anton anchored in reality.

During the periods when Anton was feeling a little better, the therapist felt more confident and allowed Anton to symbolize his inner life freely in imaginative, dramatic and free-ranging stories.

During such a good period, Anton said that there was a new pupil in his class. His name was Larry. One half of his face was blue, he had two arms plus a little arm. He had pointed ears and he kept trying to follow Anton after school. Anton said that he had struck Larry and that he would like to kill him.

The next time Anton came to the clinic he wanted to continue talking about Larry. Anton described Larry more or less in the same way as the previous week, but with a few more abnormal body parts. Larry now had one eye he could take out plus an extra leg, which made three arms and three legs, pointed ears, one eye like a telescope and one half of his face was blue. Anton claimed that Larry really existed and looked just like he had drawn him. Anton still wanted to kill Larry.

When Anton drew Larry, the third leg became an elongated penis. On the picture Anton wrote that "Larry must die". Then he rubbed the red crayon over Larry's stomach. Larry was bleeding from an arrow in his stomach. Then he drew bolts of lightening over the picture.

The reason Larry had to die was that he looked different. He had no right to exist when he looked so different. When we talked about the long penis hanging between Larry's legs, Anton said that it was a fake penis that could be pulled out.

Now the shame was captured in a picture. Now it was possible for Anton to get a handle on it.

Anton complained that Larry was spiteful. Once when he was sitting on a jetty, Larry came up from behind and pushed him down into the cold water. The water wasn't deep there. When Anton got up he saw Larry run away. The reason Larry had pushed Anton into the lake was revenge for bad thoughts. Larry knew that Anton wanted to kill him.

"With his telescope eye Larry can see what people are thinking."

Anton drew a new picture of Larry. Now Larry's penis was gone, his ears weren't pointed anymore. Larry was bleeding from an arrow that had been shot into his stomach. His eyes were angry because he was angry at Anton.

Anton got up from the chair where he had been sitting and drawing and walked up to a man-sized stuffed bear and punched it with his fist.

The therapist suggested that the bear should represent Larry. Anton started pounding the bear harder. The bear fell over and Anton pummelled it over both the head and body. Anton got very excited and he began to sexualize his actions with the bear, pinching it where its penis should have been. Then he kicked the bear in the crotch. When he was exhausted he tweaked the bear's nose and started hitting it in the head once again.

After his outburst Anton was sweaty and tired, but quite calm. The therapist praised him, because now he had truly shown his strength and his ability to direct it at someone he disliked.

After this release of pent-up tension, Anton started talking about how sad he felt when he thought of his father, who had abused him sexually and abandoned him.

During the subsequent therapy sessions, Anton wanted to continue to "kill Larry". The big bear took a lot of punishment, but the sexualized behaviour during the fights lessened more and more.

Suddenly Anton didn't want to fight with the bear anymore. He said he had become friends with Larry. Anton thought Larry was a pretty nice guy now and besides he felt sorry for Larry. And he also showed clearly that he understood that Larry didn't really exist, but represented something else. He said:

"It's not reality, it's a feeling I'm describing."

Then he drew a new picture of Larry which he called: "Larry may live."

Anton spent one whole term working out his relationship with Larry. What was the meaning of Anton's behaviour? Our interpretation was that Anton had projected his own feeling of being deviant and repulsive onto Larry. Saying that Larry should be killed was a manifestation of Anton's own self-contempt. The reconciliation with Larry was a reconciliation with himself and his own self-image. In Larry, Anton exposed a layer of shame which was processed and paled in reconciliation.

16. If you promise to be good, I suppose I can come and visit you

Frans was seven years old and had been beaten and subjected to sadistic sexual abuse by his father, who was both criminal and alcoholic. It was when he drank that he beat and sexually abused the boy. He also beat his wife. When he was sober he was nice. After many terrifying and life-threatening fights, Frans's mother had succeeded in breaking up with his father.

Now Frans hadn't seen his father for a year. Sometimes at night he dreamt that his father would come back home. With an axe in his hand he would break down the front door and when he got into the flat he would chop up both the mother and Frans himself.

At the same time Frans was afraid of his father, he missed him a great deal. He had also been a nice father, a father who had taught him to ride a bike and done fun things with him. When Frans longed for his father he became angry with his mother who wouldn't allow him to meet his father. Then he felt sorry for his father, who lived alone and wasn't allowed to see his children.

Frans was especially angry with his mother at Christmas time. Then he thought about the presents his father had undoubtedly bought for him but couldn't give to him. His simultaneous yearning for and fear of his father was a constant dilemma for Frans.

LETTER TO DADDY

On this particular day in the therapy room, Frans had written a letter to his father. In the letter he wrote:

"If you promise to be good, I suppose I can come and visit you."

The therapist suggested that Frans should post the letter in the therapy room. Frans built a house of mattresses and cushions. In the house he placed a large teddy-bear representing his father. He also built a mailbox. Under the boy's direction the therapist became a postman, who posted the letter and delivered it to Frans's father. When his father had opened the letter and read it, according to Frans he said:

"Goddamn kid!"

Then the letter exploded. There was a letter bomb in the letter, he said. Frans shrieked "Bang! Bang!" and threw himself over his father's house and destroyed it. Then he took the daddy-bear and hit it with the shaft of a floorball stick. He hit and hit until he was completely exhausted. Now his father was dead. Then he dug a grave and buried the teddy-bear. Now his father didn't exist anymore.

Suddenly there was a change of scene. Frans turned himself into an American Indian. He dressed himself in an Indian outfit and armed himself with a sword. A hostile tribe had captured his father. Now he went out on an expedition to rescue his father, who was tied up by the other Indian tribe. After a battle he managed to rescue him. He went and fetched the daddy-bear and started talking intimately with it about how he had been doing in school and about excursions they could go on together.

TURNING ONE DADDY INTO TWO

In the child's inner world the abuser can, if it is a person with whom the child has a close relation, be two persons: One whom the child likes and longs for, and one with whom the child is angry and wants to be protected from.

It may even happen that sexually abused children seek protection and solace with the very person who abused them. This transformation of a significant closely-related person to "the other", the abuser, has been experienced and attested to by many abused children. There is a risk that people close to the child are only capable of seeing one of the two, either the "good daddy" who is free of any suspicion of abuse, or the "bad daddy" who has forever forfeited the right to contact with his child.

The therapist may be inclined to "take over" the view of the abuser held by the care-giving people around the child. Not infrequently, the abuser is viewed among these people as a purely evil person. We must be aware of this tendency so that such a negative picture doesn't prevent us from seeing the child's longing for the abuser. Children need to identify with their parents and with the other significant adults around them. The child doesn't automatically identify less with the dysfunctional parent. The child continues to cling desperately to the person it is dependent on, no matter how imperfect and weak that person may be.

POSITIVE MEMORIES IMPORTANT

We consider it to be important that the child should not be deprived of its right to keep its positive memories of the abuser. It is these memories that may be the child's mental salvation when the time comes for it to form its identity. If the abuser, as in Frans's case, is the father and has been only bad, who then does the child have to turn to as a male role-model? And what kind of mother does he have who once upon a time chose to marry and have children with this bad daddy?

Alice Miller (1993) has described how a total lack of tenderness and constant cruelty on the part of a father can cause a hatred to grow in the child. "It's different for children with fathers who sometimes have fits of rage but in between these occasions are kind and happy and play with them." She takes Hitler's childhood as an example:

> *Young Adolf knew that the abuse would continue. No matter what he did, the daily beatings continued. The only option remaining was for him to deny the pain, and thereby deny himself and identify with his attacker.*

But this effect, that the child identifies with the attacker, can also be strengthened by the way the people close to the child react. There is a risk that the care-giving adults around a sexually abused child will project their own hatred of the abusing parent onto the child. The child is then at risk of denying his own good experiences of the abusing parent.

The total denunciation and vilification of the abuser by the persons close to the child can then have a reverse effect. The risk increases that the child will identify with the abuser and incorporate the abuser's pattern of behaviour.

THE HIDDEN PHOTO ALBUM

To long for, search for and be allowed to keep the bright and positive images of a father who has committed sexual abuse may take highly concrete expressions. When Uno, eight years old, and Emma, five, were alone they would look for the photo album they knew their mother had hidden behind the books in the bookcase. It contained pictures of the family and their father from the time before his sexual abuse of both children was disclosed.

It was not explicitly forbidden for them to look at these pictures, but they had received a clear message from the mother that they shouldn't like to look at them. So when she came upon them looking in the photo album once, they quickly shut it, put it back on the shelf and went away shamefaced.

In family therapy sessions following this event their mother gradually came to understand how important the positive images of their father were for the children. Even if she couldn't stand to think of him as anything but a deceitful and treacherous monster, it wasn't in the long-term best interests of the children for her to take such a one-sided view.

TWO DADDIES — A DILEMMA

Dealing with two images of the same father is a dilemma, especially in the treatment of small children. Does the child have a nice daddy who sometimes does bad things? Or a bad daddy who sometimes does nice things? The therapeutic dilemma is finding an explanation which the child can accept and which simultaneously facilitates a constructive processing of the abuse.

One way for the child to reduce its confusion when faced with the incomprehensible fact that a beloved parent has sexually abused it is simply to create two daddies. At the Boys' Clinic we affirm and reinforce this splitting of the father image. The children often display relief when we say: "When you talk about your daddy it seems as if you had not one daddy but two."

With Frans we used the concepts "nice daddy" and "bad daddy". We let both Frans and his mother talk about things the nice daddy had done and about things the bad daddy had done. We helped the mother to explain to Frans that she couldn't allow him to see his father since they could never know when he would be transformed from the nice to the bad daddy.

In Frans's case, we were able to work well with the mother. But as therapists we are not infrequently faced with a situation where the non-abusing parent finds it very difficult to accept this splitting in two that is so real to the child. Out of loyalty to the non-abusing parent the child may sometimes go along with "sacrificing" one of the two father images, assuming the father is the abuser.

Does the child become more confused and divided when we emphasize the two sides of the abuser by splitting one daddy into two? We don't think so. It is the father's split personality we are clarifying for the child. Moreover, we are creating a picture of the father that it is possible to talk about. When we say there are two daddies, the child knows that there is really only one daddy. But we can play creative games around this picture. This enables the child, in the therapy room at any rate, to destroy the bad daddy and still keep and identify with the nice daddy. Then the child can also understand why his mother chose to live with the person who became the his father, only later to turn bad and sexually abuse him.

For he was another person as well, one who was kind.

17. Catching the queer bug

— ABOUT FEAR OF BECOMING HOMOSEXUAL

Thomas said that his father had died in a fire before he himself was born. Tomas knew what he looked like because he had a photo of his father that he looked at now and then. It was a good likeness, thought Tomas, who was fourteen years old.

"My father was a cook, and that's what I'm going to be as well," said Tomas.

Conny worked on the staff of the youth recreation centre where Tomas spent a lot of time. Conny was around 30 and very popular with the kids. He was a rough-and-tumble type who liked to "roughhouse" with the boys, tackle, fight and wrestle.

One evening when Tomas and Conny were the last ones left at the centre and were helping each other to close up, Conny started roughhousing with Tomas. They wrestled and were having fun as usual when Tomas noticed that Conny had his hand up against Tomas's penis. Tomas thought it was a mistake at first, that Conny had accidentally touched him there. But Conny didn't remove his hand, and at the same time he held Tomas, "hugged" him, with the other arm. Tomas wanted Conny to stop, and tried to get loose, but Conny just laughed. And he held onto him as if they were still wrestling. Tomas noticed he was getting an erection and was ashamed of it. He said:

"Quit it!"

But Conny just kept on laughing and said:

"What do you mean, quit it? You don't seem to mind, it's just for fun."

Tomas thought Conny would get angry if he started screaming or resisting violently, so he grew still and let Conny have his way. Conny opened Tomas's trousers and masturbated him until he ejaculated. Then Conny wanted Tomas to do the same to him, but Tomas refused. He went home.

Tomas was ashamed of what Conny had done to him and didn't dare tell anyone about it. Tomas wondered why Conny had picked just him? Was Conny gay, and did he think Tomas was too? Tomas thought that he might "go queer" now that he had been "jerked off by a queer".

But Tomas kept on going to the centre, even though he knew Conny was there. The centre was his second home and Conny had always been a good guy, in spite of what had happened.

FELT FORCED

Some time later it happened again that Conny wrestled down Tomas and masturbated him. But this time Tomas didn't dare refuse when Conny wanted Tomas to do the same to him.

"I felt forced to jerk him off, since I had let him do it to me twice, even though I thought it was disgusting and didn't want to do it," related Tomas.

After this incident, Tomas was convinced he was gay or had become gay, since he had masturbated Conny.

These thoughts tormented Tomas for nearly a whole year before it was revealed that Tomas wasn't the only one Conny had been abusing. It turned out that Tomas's best friend had been subjected to the same thing. Conny was reported and charged with sexual offences. He confessed, but said that "the boys went along with it":

"We just did it for fun – just as a lark."

When Tomas came to the Boys' Clinic he was sad, introverted and tormented by the thought that he "was queer".

"I must be since I went back, even though I knew he was there," said Tomas.

A lot of time in the conversations was taken up by Tomas examining how his longing for his father could have led him to become attached to a person such as Conny, who moreover resembled the photograph of Tomas's father. It was this longing that Conny had exploited and what had happened didn't at all have to mean that Tomas was homosexual. Furthermore, it was girls he fantasized about and yearned for, although he hadn't been together with one yet.

Tomas was plagued by nightmares where Conny came towards him, hugged him, held him fast, threatened him. He was also obsessed with thoughts of revenge. Tomas wanted to "beat Conny's brains out" and said "he ought to be burnt at the stake".

"But I don't want to become a murderer," said Tomas.

We tried to disentangle all the threads, the rage at the fact that his own father had died in a fire and the betrayal of the new father-figure Conny, who he now wished would also die in a fire (be burnt at the stake) in his fantasies.

FEAR OF BECOMING HOMOSEXUAL

Tomas shares this fear of being or becoming homosexual as a result of being sexually abused by a man with many of the boys we have come into contact with. "Catching the queer bug", as one boy put it. This is a central theme to work on, especially for the slightly older boys.

Of course, we must also be open to the possibility that some boys will become homosexuals and be careful not to make them guilty about this. Many adult men who were sexually abused as boys have attested to this confusion as to sexual affinity, regardless of whether they have been the victims of male or female abusers.

Rogers and Terry (1984) conducted a study showing that all boys who have been victims of homosexual abuse exhibited confusion and consternation regarding their sexual identity. They believe that this confusion has to do with the boys' wondering why they were "picked" by the perpetrator, their concern that the perpetrator had "discovered" a latent homosexuality in them which they themselves had not been aware of, and their inability to resist the assaults.

Against this background, Tomas appears to be very typical in his reactions.

18. Teacher's pets

— TREATMENT OF A GROUP

Seven fourteen-year-old boys had been sexually abused by a paedophile and were in therapy at the Boys' Clinic.

The background of the story was interesting. When the boys were in second grade they had a male teacher. When the children were learning sums, he moved the boys who were a little slow to learn up to the front. They had to sit on the teacher's lap and do the sums. While the boys were sitting there on his lap, he stuck his hand down their trousers and fondled their penises. The teacher's abuse was not visible to the rest of the class. The front side of his desk hid it from view.

The teacher continued his abuse for nearly two years. When one of the children broke the silence, the others came forward and revealed that they had also been molested. About ten children had been molested by the teacher.

The teacher left the school and the affair was kept quiet. No one talked with the children about their experiences. Nor was any information given out on what had happened to the teacher. Life in the school went on with a silent parenthesis around what had happened.

EXPERIENCED SCHOOL NURSE

The years passed and the boys entered seventh grade. A new, but experienced, school nurse had come to work at the school. Her duties included sex education.

The nurse had no knowledge of the affair with the teacher four years earlier. When she visited one of the seventh-grade classes she wondered why it was impossible to conduct any instruction in sexual matters in this particular class. A group of boys sabotaged the instruction completely. They sexualized wildly, screamed and wrote coarse sexual words on the walls of the school. The word "queer" recurred constantly. They hated and threatened to kill all queers.

The school nurse was used to dealing with young boys, but this group was more sexually demonstrative than she was accustomed to. She started wondering what kinds of problems the boys who were doing the worst screaming had concerning their sexuality. Instead of pushing the boys away she tried to draw them nearer. She asked them to come to her office one at a time.

With her interested and non-moralizing manner she won the boys' confidence. The group she had identified as the "troublemakers" were the very boys who had been sexually abused by the teacher. The boys told her of the anger they still carried with them towards the teacher.

The school nurse got in touch with us and the therapy work could begin.

WE AREN'T QUEERS

The boys who came to us saw gays everywhere. And gays were something they had to defend themselves against in all situations. When they met two men in the therapy room, we naturally also became gays in their eyes.

All therapeutic work with these fantasies was impossible at this stage. What the boys first needed help with was simply to sit still so we could talk to them.

We set boundaries for their fantasies by being candid about ourselves. We told them we weren't gay, that we lived in ordinary families with wives and children. That information reassured the boys.

During the initial conversation we let each one of them talk about what he remembered from the abuse. We let them describe what the classroom looked like, what the names of their classmates were, what the teacher looked like, how he abused them – everything in as much detail as possible. We tried to get them to remember how many times the teacher had fondled their penises. In short, we tried to help them talk about what had happened.

Someone also thought he had seen the teacher, who was now working as a security guard at a sports arena. We assigned them the task of finding out as much as they could about the teacher. What had happened to him, had he been convicted of any crime, where did he go?

DIRECTING ANGER

These boys, like so many of the boys who have come to us, were angry children who didn't know where to direct their anger. In the school they acted out their anger in an uncontrolled and destructive fashion. They ruined things for themselves and for others, both materially and emotionally.

Our work was to try to help these boys direct their anger and put words to it.

One day the boys made up a game where they directed their anger at the perpetrator. The game was violent, sometimes extremely so. The point was to "kill" Ben.

Ben was the name of the teacher who had perpetrated the abuse. There was a bedspread in the therapy room. The bedspread was thrown over the head of someone in the group. The one with the bedspread over him had to be Ben. One boy held the bedspread over Ben's head. The others hit him hard and brutally until he managed to twist free and throw the bedspread over the head of another member of the group. Then he became Ben.

So the bedspread flew from boy to boy. Everyone got to hit and everyone was at one time or another Ben and got beaten. Our job was to keep the game under control and help them give words to their feelings. All the time during the game the boys shrieked:

"Kill Ben! Kill Ben!"

We intervened by shouting over the general melee:

"Why must he be killed?"

Then they were able to use more words for their emotions and they shouted while they hit:

"Because you played with my willy you dirty queeeeer!"

When they had fought for about fifteen minutes we would go in and stop the "kill Ben game", which was not always easy. Fourteen-year-olds are strong. Eventually we figured out a way that worked well with the group (and might also please a certain well-known soft drink manufacturer). When we thought they had fought enough we shouted as loud as we could:

"COCA-COLA!"

That put an immediate stop to the tumult. The boys sat down in a ring and we were able to start talking with cans of coke in our hands.

We thought the "kill Ben game" contained a number of reparative components. It was creative; the boys made it up themselves. It gave them an outlet for their anger, which was directed towards the perpetrator. It also gave them an opportunity to train self-defence and learn to protect themselves against abuse. The one who got the bedspread over his head had to try to get free as quickly as possible. It had verbal components. It got the boys to put words to their anger. And it also may have enabled them to experience some empathy with the abuser, since each one got to be Ben at one time or another. The "kill Ben game" was played at the start of the group meetings for a whole term before it ended of its own accord.

EMOTIONAL TRIAL

We didn't have very great hopes when it came to getting boys in a group to express their emotions surrounding being a victim. Most boys are very reluctant to show weakness. Expressing fear means they have to lower their defences, and thereby become vulnerable. They run the risk of being teased for showing their feelings.

In actual fact, it went unexpectedly well. But we didn't press particularly hard to get the boys to open up to each other. At the same time that we accepted their own means of expression, we nevertheless tried to find suitable games that could help them to express difficult emotions, without losing face in front of their friends. One such game was "Emotional Trial".

The game was played like this: Since the boys didn't know whether Ben, the abusive teacher, had been convicted of any crime or received any punishment, we decided to hold our own trial and pass sentence. One of the therapists was picked to be the judge. The other therapist was Ben's defence attorney. A large teddy-bear was placed in a chair to be Ben. The judge started by asking the boys to tell what Ben had done to them. Then the judge turned to each of the boys and asked what penalty they thought Ben should receive. He reminded them that this was an emotional trial, and in such a trial the penalty should cause the same suffering as that experienced by the abused child.

One boy suggested that Ben should receive the death penalty. The judge asked him how he thought Ben should be executed.

"He should be killed slowly by sticking two thousand needles in his body."

"Where should the needles be stuck?"

"In the heart."

In the role play the boy communicated what he had felt when he was being abused and afterwards. He had also had difficulty sleeping when he thought about the teacher, and had been afraid of meeting him again. The judge then proposed that the penalty be broadened to include disturbing the defendant in his sleep and making him feel afraid of meeting the boy.

THE DEFENCE ATTORNEY HAS THE WORD

Then Ben's defence attorney made a plea on behalf of his client. He referred to extenuating circumstances and said that Ben wanted the boys to be good in arithmetic and that he loved the boys and didn't want to hurt them in any way. He had just thought that the boys were so nice and cute that he couldn't help fondling their willies a little. That wasn't so terrible, was it? He hadn't hurt them. During the defence plea the boys got excited and shouted:

"Damn queer! You're wrong! You have too hurt us!"

The judge banged his gavel on the table and demanded order in the court, which everyone ignored.

Another boy got to tell about how disgusted, confused and upset he had felt. He had also suffered from not being able to show how he had felt.

"What should the penalty be?" asked the judge.

They quickly arrived at the conclusion that Ben should also go around feeling disgusted, angry, confused and upset for four years without being able to show it to anyone.

And so the judge continued going through all the boys' personal sufferings. Ben's defence attorney tried to play down the events, which brought out the boys' feelings even more. After a recess the judge passed judgement and read the sentence. It was a litany of all the suffering the boys had expressed. The judge sentenced Ben to the same suffering.

After the trial the boys applauded spontaneously, were very satisfied, relaxed and natural. No tough talk, no one teased anyone else.

MEETING WITH HOMOSEXUALS

Eventually the time came to have a dialogue with the boys about homosexuality. The boys had a clear and outspoken opinion of homosexuals: Queers were people you hated and were afraid of. Queers could attack them and rape them. Quite simply, queers were people you should knock down so they couldn't rape you.

The group exploded in nervous hoots and howls when we suggested inviting a homosexual man and a homosexual woman whom the boys could interview. The idea was frightening, but eventually it also became fascinating. Preparations for the meeting took four months. We had phoned RFSL (the Swedish Federation for Gay and Lesbian Rights), which promised to send someone when the boys felt ready to receive them. The boys prepared questions which they would put to the homosexual guests.

This is how the questions to the lesbian girl were formulated:

1. How did you become lesbian?
2. What do you do when you make love?
3. Do you always have the same partner?
4. Where do you meet your partners?
5. What did your parents say?
6. Where are you when you make love?
7. How many girlfriends have you had?
8. Have you ever slept with a guy?
9. Do you have a vibrator?
10. Do you fool around a lot with yourself?
11. When did you do it the first time?
12. Do you often cheat?

The questions to the homosexual man were formulated as follows:

1. Why did you become gay?
2. When did you know that you were gay?
3. What do your parents think about the fact that you're gay?
4. Do you feel abnormal?
5. How did it feel when you went to school?
6. What does it feel like to be gay?
7. Do you go around flirting in public?
8. Do you go to gay dances?
9. Do you walk the street?
10. What do you do when you get together?
11. Is it easy to find a partner?
12. Were you afraid the first time?
13. Did it hurt?
14. Do you often masturbate?
15. What does it feel like to be butt-fucked?
16. Do you suck cock after it has been in your ass?
17. Do you poke yourself in the ass when you're horny?

When the boys had compiled the questions they became nervous. How would they ever be able to ask them when the guests were there? Our demand was that they, not we, should ask the questions.

The meeting with the homosexuals was successful beyond our expectations. The gay man was not dressed in leather as the boys had thought he would be. He looked quite ordinary.

The boys were collected, not silly. They said that they had been sexually molested by their teacher when they were in second and third grade. They said that they had prepared questions they wondered about. The boys had divided the questions up among themselves so that they didn't have to ask their own questions. This is what a question might sound like:

"Do you go to gay dances? I'm not the one who wrote this question, it's that guy over there, Jesper."

Not having to ask their own questions made the boys feel more secure.

The meeting was a turning point for the boys in terms of their attitude towards homosexuals. They asked all the questions they had prepared for the girl. They asked all the questions they had prepared for the man except the last three. We regarded excluding those questions as a sign of good judgement on the part of the boys. They began to like our guests and didn't want to get too impertinent in their questions.

During the meeting the boys found out that many gay men never have sex. They don't dare tell anyone that they're homosexual, they feel shame and they refrain from having any sexual partners. The homosexual man explained in detail what it had been like for him in school and how he came to the insight that he was a homosexual. The boys hung on his every word and asked a lot of questions.

The lesbian girl talked about herself in a personal and vivid manner. She talked, for example, about how difficult it is and how long it can take for a lesbian woman to find a sexual partner. In a man-woman relationship it is often the man who takes the initiative for sex. When it is two women who want to be with each other it can take time before either one takes the initiative.

The boys spoke for a long time afterwards about what a cool queer they had talked with. The meeting changed the boys' attitudes toward homosexuals. Their fear and hostility toward gays diminished considerably. It actually diminished so much that we didn't notice it anymore.

We don't think we could have brought about the same attitude changes by talking about homosexuals as by talking with them.

The boys were in therapy for three terms. They came every fourteen days. During the last term the conversationsmainly revolved around normal adolescent subjects: relationships with girls, school, how they could repair their reputations as rowdies and cut-ups in school.

When we look back on this work we think that the sexual abuse was processed in a reasonable fashion. It was described and made real, a direction was found for the anger, feelings came out, attitudes towards homosexuals were re-examined. The boys' normal teenage speculations about sex and interpersonal relations and about themselves were also given plenty of room.

19. Sex ring

When a paedophile is exposed, it is the rule rather than the exception that he has abused more than one child. Often it turns out that he is a member of a paedophilic sex ring.

The most common type of sex ring is when a male paedophile abuses a group of boys. But there may also be several abusers, either several male paedophiles who work together, or both male and female abusers working together.

MULTI-FAMILY MEETING

Furniss (1991) believes that the first thing that should be done when a sex ring has been discovered is to organize a multi-family meeting. The meeting needs to be attended by all children who have been abused as well as their parents. In addition, the child welfare authorities should be present, as well as the police officer in charge of the investigation, if possible. The presence of the police officer can be of great therapeutic value, since he or she can give a factual account of the abusive offences. The police account helps the family get an overall picture of the abuse.

The aim of the multi-family meeting is to inform everyone of all the factual details concerning what happened in the sex ring and to help the families find a language for communicating thoughts and feelings both between different sets of parents and between children and parents. A multi-family meeting is a good starting point for subsequent treatment.

Important topics during the multi-family meeting are:

1. Can the parents believe that the sex ring actually existed?
2. Can they believe that their own child has been part of the ring and has been sexually abused?
3. What do they feel about the fact that the abuse has happened right under their noses?
4. What do they feel about their own child having been abused?
5. What do they feel about their child not having told them?
6. Does anyone blame the child for the abuse?
7. How does the abuse affect their sense of control and their ability to parent?
8. In what ways do the parents feel they are in the same situation or in a different situation compared with other parents?
9. Do the mothers feel the same as the fathers about what has happened? What are the differences and the similarities?

OUR EXPERIENCE

We have tested this model at the Boys' Clinic and found it to be both valuable and problematic. The most valuable part has been the questions recommended by Furniss for the multi-family meeting.

For us, however, it was difficult to assemble all the parents to more than one multi-family meeting. Fewer and fewer parents showed up at each new meeting. The parents thought the first meeting was good, but then they preferred to come one at a time.

Bringing all the children who have been victims in a sex ring together also proved difficult. The children don't always know each other. The abuser may have met children in different contexts where the children had no mutual knowledge of each other. This becomes a complicating factor. Children who have been abused are extremely afraid of it becoming known in school and of being teased for being homosexuals. A sense of complicity is greater among children who have been abused by paedophiles who have not been violent and who have not threatened them. They are

118

therefore afraid to talk about the abuse with other children, even if they have experienced the same things and are just as scared themselves.

Perhaps a more fruitful treatment strategy is to divide the sex ring victims into smaller groups. Then the children who know each other from before and have had the secret about the abuse in common can process the events.

In one sex ring case we were involved with, the perpetrator had both filmed and photographed his own acts of abuse. This led to his conviction in court. But it was also a serious problem for both the children and the parents.

How was the evidence being stored? Who had seen it? Who had access to it? Should the children be allowed to see it? These were some of the questions posed at the therapy meetings.

Another observation we made was that very few fathers came to the multi-family meetings. And for each new meeting, fewer and fewer fathers came.

Naturally the parents are important in conjunction with the disclosure that a child has been abused. In our experience the feelings and reactions of siblings are equally important. There is a risk that a sibling may tease and lay blame if the siblings are not invited to participate in at least part of the therapy.

To the extent that "our" boys have been teased for being "queer" or suchlike following paedophilic abuse, the teasing has been done by unsympathetic siblings who may have thought that "it's your own fault since you went there".

The emotions that have been expressed in our parent groups have been complex and heated. The parents have accused themselves of being bad parents for not realizing what was going on. They have blamed the children for not telling. Some fathers have wanted to take justice into their own hands and planned violent revenge.

And all have felt betrayed and tricked by someone they have trusted, since the paedophile had been in touch with the families and gained their confidence in order to gain access to the children. Concern about the children's future, their sexual identity and possible damage has also been ventilated in the parent groups.

20. Daddy's in a coffin on the couch

— A CASE DESCRIPTION

THE FIRST MONTH

Matthew, nine years old, came to the Boys' Clinic with his mother. They had travelled a long way, several hours by train. The boy was afraid of his father, afraid he would come back home again, get violent and dangerous like he had been before. His mother was also afraid, but with time her anger had come to dominate her fear. She was angry because she was afraid and because of what he had done to her son. She was also self-reproachful. She thought she ought to have stopped the father's sadistic attacks earlier.

The father had beaten the mother when Matthew was very small. At first the father got violent when he was drunk, but with time he also got violent when he was sober.

Matthew's father hit him for the first time when he was two years old. The violence was repeated. When the police came, the father used Matthew as a shield and threatened to kill Matthew if they tried to arrest him. The mother should have left him then and there, she thought. But she didn't. He was allowed to come home again and the violence continued for five more years.

Matthew related frightening memories. His father had forced Matthew to undress and then held his penis. Then Matthew had been forced to hold his father's penis. Then his father had lifted him out through the window on the third floor and said he would drop him if he told anyone. His father had also forced Matthew to use oral snuff and drink alcohol. He had forced him to watch pornographic and violent movies.

Matthew's most frightening memory was when his father had been drunk and locked himself in a room with Matthew. There his father had pointed a gun at him. Matthew thought he was going to die. After that event, Matthew started to eat compulsively.

"I ate away my fear."

Matthew became an overweight child. He suffered from stomach pains.

"It feels like I'm being kicked in the stomach. Then I have to sit down with a pillow pressed against my stomach until it goes away."

Usually he got a stomachache in the morning when he had to go to school. Matthew also had difficulty sleeping. He seldom fell asleep before midnight. In the evenings he was hungry.

"I eat until I'm full, then I get hungry again."

His mother tried to stop his overeating, but failed.

At the Boys' Clinic Matthew wanted to draw. One picture showed how his mother and little brother are sitting on a couch, he is standing off to the side and his father is lying in a coffin on the couch. Another picture showed him watching a violent film on television with his father.

At home he wanted to build with lego and watch television. His mother worried that Matthew had no friends.

Comments

Matthew was caught in a vicious circle; the more he ate the less afraid he felt. But the price for alleviating the fear was that he got fat and clumsy, felt different and isolated himself more. His morning stomachache gave him a legitimate reason to stay home from school and avoid feeling inferior.

His mother's difficulties in breaking the vicious circle are easy to understand. In the first place, her son had experienced some terrible things, and in the second place she felt guilty for not having stopped the abuse earlier.

Handling conflicts with a child that has been having a tough time, for which you feel partly to blame, is a complicated matter. Matthew therefore came to exercise power and control at home in a destructive manner. By wielding that power he compensated for the powerlessness he felt within himself. But this compensation led him backward, not forward.

LOSS OF HEARING

When we asked Matthew if there was anything he hadn't told us he suddenly suffered a loss of hearing. He didn't hear the question. When we repeated the question he cupped his hand behind his ear and strained to hear.

His mother explained that Matthew had trouble hearing sometimes. She had also had the same problem when she was a child. The mother's hearing had deteriorated to the point where she got a hearing aid. When she had got the hearing aid, her hearing problem disappeared and she never had to use it. Matthew had trouble hearing when he was asked about his father's abuse of him. He also had difficulty remaining seated in the chair. On one occasion he went limp and slid off the chair into a little heap on the floor when we brought up the subject of his father. When we changed the subject and started drawing rebuses and giving him funny riddles, he woke up and could hear again.

Comments:

The boy's hearing loss and sudden limpness when we spoke about his father is an example of dissociation. We interpret this as indicating that this was how he had dealt with the frightening abuse situations he had experienced with his father. Matthew developed the same symptom his mother had had when she was small, loss of hearing. His mother had also been an incest victim. She was also raised in a chaotic home with drunkenness and violence. Shutting off her hearing may have been the only way she had of protecting herself.

THIRD MONTH

It was difficult for Matthew to talk about his fear and it was difficult for him to play in the playroom at the Boys' Clinic. It took a long time before he got up the courage to start using the play materials. One day he drew a nasty figure holding a bottle and a knife. It was his father. Matthew said he had seen his father scare a boy with the knife. He didn't know for sure if the blood came from the boy or if his father had cut himself by accident.

"The boy ran away," said Matthew.

"It's good that he ran. It may be best if you banish your daddy to a safe place," said the therapist.

"To hell, let him roast in hell!" said Matthew.

RED CUSHIONS IN HELL

Matthew started building a hell in the playroom.

"There should be red cushions," said Matthew.

Our big rubber ball, which looks like a goat with its horns, was naturally given the role of the Devil. It was placed in hell. The drawing of Matthew's father was also placed in hell. The Devil started to eat the father. Matthew got a fork and let the Devil stick holes in his drawing with it. Then he let the Devil keep the cut-up drawing of his father in the "larder".

When his father had been put away in the Devil's larder, Matthew put on his boxing gloves and started punching the therapist until he got tired. Then he went to the table and drank juice and caught his breath. Matthew looked relieved and relaxed. When he had got his breath back he wanted to build a paradise. There were to be yellow cushions there. A cat was placed in the paradise. The therapist asked if the Devil was allowed to come visit in paradise. The Devil was absolutely forbidden to come there. If he did he would be attacked by a ball that sprayed water.

"If the Devil comes to paradise it will burn up," said Matthew.

The session ended when Matthew fetched his mother from the waiting room and had a picnic with her in paradise.

At our next meeting the mother said that Matthew had gone home and torn down a lego wall he had built in the room to divide off the evil and dangerous half of the room from the good and safe half. Now he had taken control of his entire room.

Comments

The boy handed his father over to the Devil. But the father wasn't executed. The Devil was going to keep him in his larder. The fact that the father was to be spared we took as an expression of hope that the father would be able to return some day as a reformed person. As long as Matthew was afraid of his father, he would have to be kept prisoner in the Devil's larder. After he had built the hell in our playroom and consigned the evil person he was afraid of to that place, he didn't need the lego wall in his room at home anymore. The evil person was safely stored away in the hell at the Boys' Clinic.

FIFTH MONTH

Now Matthew wanted to fight every time. His stomachache was gone. He ate less and had lost weight. He vented his aggression on the rubber ball with horns. He failed with a drawing. That was the rubber ball's fault. Now it was going to get beaten for ten thousand years. With a sword it would only take six thousand years.

Matthew wanted to wrestle with the therapist. When he had punched and wrestled himself util he was tired he wanted his mother to come in from the waiting room. He wanted her to draw a tree. He complimented his mother for making such a nice drawing. He took the tree home to put up on his wall. Before he went home he hugged the therapist and said: "Now I'm going to faint" and went limp.

Comments:

Now Matthew had become less afraid. He had begun to direct his anger outwards. We assume that Matthew, like other sexually abused children, also harboured anger towards the non-abusing parent. We also assume that such feelings of anger towards the mother were frightening for him. After all, his mother was the only security he had. Asking his mother to draw a tree, something which is firmly rooted in the ground, something that is always there, was perhaps an expression of a desire that his mother would always be there for him, and at the same time an attempt to stem his angry feelings towards her. Matthew's limp hugs were touching and painful. In them he showed clearly his longing for tenderness and at the same time the fact that he had never been allowed to show this need for tenderness to his father.

Both Matthew and his mother were each instructed to make their own drawing. Matthew drew a planet with people who spoke a secret language and lived underground.

His mother drew a planet where the people were nice and lived on the surface. There was a school, nice people and tame animals. The people who lived underground on Matthew's planet wanted to get in touch with the mother's planet. But they couldn't because her planet had a different atmosphere.

"The radio waves can't get through," said Matthew.

The atmosphere around Matthew's planet was evil and consisted of all the wicked souls. Suddenly the mother understood that Matthew was trying to reach her but was unable to. She drew an apparatus that could receive the evil waves and turn them off. In that way the underground creatures with the secret language on Matthew's planet could come to the mother's planet and go to "peace school".

"But if the secret gets out, they would be afraid of visits by scientists and shut themselves in for another two hundred years," said Matthew.

Comments:

Were there other things that had happened but had not been told? Were the things that hadn't been told secret or forgotten?

On Matthew's planet, the inhabitants lived underground and had a secret language. What was Matthew trying to express when he asked: "If the secret gets out, they would shut themselves in for another two hundred years"? A long time. Were "scientists" therapists? Didn't Matthew want to reveal more about nasty things he had experienced, or were there other secrets? Secrets he was afraid would destroy his mother and himself if they were revealed? The safest thing was perhaps to have them locked up.

FOURTEENTH MONTH

Matthew played with the spider game, where you have to rescue insects who are stuck in a spider web. Now he was going to rescue his mother who had got stuck in the web. Then he wanted to teach the therapist jujitsu holds, which he had learned in a self-defence course. Matthew had nothing to talk about.

This time the mother was with them in the therapy room and she wanted them to talk about how Matthew was behaving towards his little brother. He had started frightening him and calling him dirty names such as "queer" and "cock". On the metro he had shouted "queer" at his little brother. His mother had become so angry that she had tweaked Matthew's nose.

Matthew didn't want to talk about this. He preferred to stand in the window and throw himself down on the cushions. The therapist laid two mattresses under the cushions so that Matthew wouldn't hurt himself. With the sword in his hand, Matthew dived from the window down onto the cushions. It was a high jump. The therapist suggested that Matthew should say angry things to his little brother during the time he was in the air. But he wasn't allowed to say queer or cock. Matthew said:

"Bad Carl! Damn Carl! Bonehead! Stupid Carl! Stop that! Naughty Carl!"

Matthew liked the game. He thought it was fun to see how many words he could manage to say while he was in the air. The therapist was also satisfied. He had affirmed Matthew's play initiative, but added a space where Matthew could put new words to his anger, or perhaps his jealousy, towards his little brother. In the air between the window and the floor he could do this.

Comments:
Matthew started finding new strategies to feel big and invulnerable. His little brother was an easy target. When he scared his little brother, Matthew transferred his own fear and helplessness onto him. Diving from the window became yet another proof of Matthew's strength. In this way he showed that he had become more agile and less clumsy since he had cut down on his eating. The therapist did not wish to interfere with such a new defence. The new behaviour had, after all, given him new freedom. It had in turn reduced his fear. Even if his newly-found freedom wasn't altogether functional, it was better than being afraid.

Naturally his little brother had to be protected. Matthew didn't question his mother's tweaking his nose.

TWENTIETH MONTH

Our next theme was to see if we could raise Matthew's self-confidence, help him to find situations where he could feel good and help him to see himself as a normal and fairly successful boy, despite his partially unhappy childhood. His mother decided to transfer him to an ordinary school class. Matthew was attending a small, special class for children with special needs. The objective of the sessions now was that Matthew should be made as comfortable as possible; be pleased with himself. We devoted hours to making things as pleasant as possible, guessing riddles, telling stories, playing games. Matthew nudged and shoved a lot and liked body contact consisting of pushes mixed with hugs. The therapist noted the strong yearning for a father that Matthew had inside him.

Comments:

Children have a natural need to get on with their lives and put the past behind them. The therapeutic challenge is to get the child to stop short, to start remembering and feeling. But when this has been accomplished and the child has indeed stopped short, we must also be able to help it to build up some kind of workable defences. We believe that remaining occupied for years with past sexual abuse can inhibit the child's ability to build new constructive defences around the painful events of the past. We thought we were approaching the time for a conclusion with Matthew.

TWENTY-THIRD MONTH

The concluding session. Matthew's mother and little brother participated for a while. The mother said that Matthew was going to change schools and attend a normal class next term. She thought that would be better for Matthew. When his mother and little brother had left, Matthew and the therapist went out and rented a video. Munching on crisps and sweets, they sat together and watched the film.

Nothing much was said.

21. My child was a monster

– A MOTHER'S STORY

When you have all the facts in hand and know that sexual abuse has occurred, it is easy in retrospect to see all the signs and signals that something wasn't right. But when you're in the midst of the process, it isn't at all as simple to see what is going on. In this chapter we shall describe how things may appear from a mother's point of view in this situation.

Mari was a single mother to Nicklas, age seven. To give Mari some relief and enable her to study, Mari's former boyfriend Leif had been assigned by the local social services department as a contact man for Nicklas. Nicklas stayed with Leif regularly over a period of about four years. Eventually it came out that Nicklas had been sexually abused from the time he was two until he was six.

We would like to try here to give a picture of Mari's feelings, thoughts and observations from the time she first began to suspect that Leif had perhaps done something with Nicklas until she broke up with Leif, and Nicklas eventually began to tell what had happened.

Mari is not an unusual mother. The inability and reluctance to acknowledge what she actually saw, to comprehend what she really knew, is something she shares with many other parents in the same situation.

But this story is also about a boy who tries to show that something is wrong, but who is unable to articulate it in words. The symptoms these boys display with their behaviour and acting-out can many times be extremely provocative.

This is how it was for Mari:

I know that I thought that Nicklas was simply an out-and-out monster. In every way, through and through, all the time, about everything. I couldn't do anything without there being something that he could manufacture a problem from, even though everything might be great. Everything was so upside-down.

There was nothing I could do to be a good mother. No matter whether I scolded him and set firm limits, and was really picky, or whether I tried to coax or talk, nothing I did was right.

I thought it had to do with the fact that I was a single parent and had worked a great deal. Then when I went back to school, he had longer days at the day nursery than ever before. And then I thought it had to do with his father, who had no contact with us, or that Leif was so bad at setting limits, since he was always extra difficult when he'd been staying with him.

Mari's very first memory of suspecting that something was wrong is when a guest lecturer at her school talked about sexual abuse.

I felt really bad when she was talking. I didn't recognize myself, since I'm accustomed to hearing all kinds of things. It was so strange and I didn't know how I was going to get through that afternoon. I cried in the car and had to muster all my strength to dry away my tears so I could get home. This feeling of anxiety just flooded over me.

The feeling stayed with me for several days. I wondered what it was all about. I thought maybe it was something in me, something I had been through myself. I went to a therapist who worked with hypnosis. No, she didn't think that was the case.

After the lecture I started putting two and two together. And slowly but surely – at first I didn't dare face head-on what it was really all about – I started to put the pieces of the puzzle together.

Those strange photographs that Leif had taken. I think there were two, showing the same thing, one was more intimate. Nicklas was lying and sleeping with his legs curled up, they were taken from the behind with the cover pulled down and he didn't have any trousers on.

On the one that was more of a close-up you could see his penis and his scrotum, and I thought it was a disgusting picture. I showed it to a friend, then I tore it up and threw it away. The other one I was also going to tear up, but I didn't want to do it right away since I thought Nicklas would get really angry if he discovered I had taken his photo. Then I forgot it, luckily.

But there were other pieces to the puzzle. Nicklas masturbated frequently and furiously in a way that was hardly natural.

It was in the bathroom when he was going to get dressed or undressed, he would just sit there and get stuck in there. He was very rough, he pulled hard on his penis. I said to him: "Be careful of your penis, you only have one."

Then he started hiding. He built a fort and hid inside it and I wasn't allowed to disturb him. But I got real curious, so I tried to find an excuse to go in, and then he got really angry.

Towards the end he masturbated more or less every day. He did it all the time, it seemed. Later he told me how he would stick a finger or a pencil up his bottom, like Leif did with him. Then he stuck small cannon-balls from a toy cannon under his foreskin. He could play with himself for a long time, half an hour, an hour. He also tried to rub his penis against me and French-kiss, even in front of our friends.

What was it about Leif that Mari had been fond of, that brought them together in the first place? Did she notice anything about his relationship with Nicklas or anything special about Leif himself that she can understand better now? We go back a little in time.

Leif seemed kind and timid. He felt solid, and he came from the West Coast just like me, liked the ocean and all that.

He played with Nicklas from the start and was very straightforward in his contact with him. It was great to meet a man who liked children so much, I thought, being a single mother. He told me himself that he fell for me because of Nicklas, and I thought he was really anxious to have a child.

131

*But it was impossible to have sex with him. I think that's rather
essential. He never managed to get an erection one single time when
we went to bed with each other.*

Leif was appointed to be Nicklas' contact person.

*I don't know exactly the right words, but I do know a feeling I had that
was very clear. It was: Okay, now I've been really rotten to you, you
poor guy. I broke up with you, you who've had a tough time in life.
You've hardly had a girl all your life, but okay, I'll let you take care of
my child.*

*I know that I hadn't thought that thought in such explicit terms,
but I know it was there all the same. Some kind of guilt towards him.
Since they had such a good relationship, and he was such a father
figure, and since Nicklas didn't have a father, why couldn't he be
Nicklas's contact person?*

The change in Nicklas came gradually, and the situation grew worse and
worse.

*I tried desperately to straighten out our lives, which were all
topsy-turvy. We quarrelled almost all the time, and Nicklas often hurt
me, hit me, jumped on me. Once he tried to stick a pencil in my eye,
another time he threatened me with a pair of scissors.*

*We never had any rest, and sometimes I hit him, to my own
horror. And I yelled a lot at Nicklas.*

*But at the same time I kept trying to find ways to reach him
through play, reading, small talk. Sometimes we got along well
together for a while, but suddenly he would fly into a rage for no
reason or ruin things in some way. It was like climbing a hill that just
got higher and higher.*

Mari's suspicions were aroused and she started putting her puzzle together.

*During this "putting-the-puzzle-together" period it was as if I was
holding my breath. I didn't want to believe, but something was driving
me forward since I didn't want to leave the matter without examining*

it. But I didn't believe it. I didn't want to believe it. I had big blinders on. I checked and I phoned, I read and I worried and I spoke with friends and asked if they had noticed anything about Nicklas.

And they had. When Nicklas had slept over at the neighbour's and changed clothes in the evening, he had lain on his back and very deliberately displayed his bottom. The mother had reacted to this.

Someone else had seen how Leif, at a children's party, sought out the company of the children, had difficulty sitting and talking to adults. Then a mother had seen how he stroked her son's arm in a way she didn't like. They had never met before. On that occasion she had thought, well, maybe he is a homosexual even though he doesn't know it.

I actually understood, but I just couldn't take it in. It became so clear when I put all the pieces of the puzzle together that it was just too much to be a coincidence.

The staff at the day nursery hadn't actually noticed anything concrete, but they had reacted to the fact that Nicklas had withdrawn more and more into his shell during the past few years. And he did have relational problems. He didn't know how to play with other children. During one period he had just run around, and then just kissed, and then just tickled. During another period he had gone in for scaring the other children.

So it took a long time for me to open my eyes. It took me three months from my first suspicions to when I began to comprehend what was going on.

But I didn't know what to do and I was still not completely sure, couldn't quite believe it was true.

At first Mari wanted to confront Leif with her suspicions.

I told Leif that he couldn't set limits. Furthermore he was always giving Nicklas gifts. I told him this just couldn't continue, my relationship with Nicklas is so chaotic, you have to stop giving him presents.

Nicklas had begun doing what many sexually abused children do. He tried to find a way to tell, to see if his mother was capable of receiving what he carried within him but was incapable of saying out loud.

> *In the evenings Nicklas wanted me to play a game with him that he had made up himself. He called it "Say hello to Josefin". Josefin lived on Nicklas's back. I was supposed to walk with my fingers along his back and ask him how Josefin was, since she knew everything about Nicklas. Josefin took me to an attic where there was an old trunk with letters telling all about Nicklas and how he was doing. To get into the attic I needed a special key. But the key was lost and the trunk had to be broken open. But when we were going to read the letters, it turned out they were so old and faded that all the words had disappeared. All you could see was: Help, help...*
>
> *It was extremely painful for I understood that he wanted to tell me something but that he couldn't get the words out.*

Another sign was that Nicklas's bottom had been red on several occasions. And Mari had seen a connection. She let Nicklas visit Leif one last time to have her suspicions finally confirmed.

> *It was very difficult. I was torn in two trying to make up my mind. I felt that since there wasn't any definite proof, this was the way to get it. I sent Nicklas there one last time because I had realized the connection between the red bottom and the stays with Leif. But since I wasn't completely sure, I took the chance to get evidence, and it turned out I was right. So I don't regret it. Without that proof I probably wouldn't have dared to stand firm in my search for help in the way I was now able to. You don't accuse someone of sexual abuse without being very, very certain.*
>
> *I can't say I regret that I did it. I feel so sick at having sent him to Leif so many other times without realizing anything, so one more time I don't think makes any difference. After all, I did it because I had to have some positive proof to go on. I think it was good in some strange way, even though he was definitely abused that time as well.*

Mari got her proof. And yet it didn't all turn out the way she had hoped.

Nicklas said to me the next morning: "No, nothing happened to me at Leif's, you have to believe me, mummy". He stuck to his story without flinching. That made me confused.

After that Mari finally ended her relationship with Leif. And life for Mari and Nicklas entered a new phase.

Very soon after the break Nicklas started telling me what a good mother I was "because you do such good things". He started drawing hearts and writing "I love you" over and over, constant declarations of love. The difference was so striking. And at the day nursery he had started painting in colours he had never used before, it was as if something had been set free inside him so that he could finally tell.

We had also continued playing "Say hello to Josefin". The letters in the trunk become more and more legible, and late on the first evening of summer vacation, when he knew we would be together all summer, Nicklas couldn't sleep. He came down the stairs in his pyjamas and asked if it was because of those pictures that he wasn't allowed to see Leif anymore. And then he started to tell me what Leif had done, about the willy game and the bottom game, about all the "why questions" he had had in his head all the time but hadn't dared to talk about because then he would get a smacking.

That's how it started. It was obvious he really wanted to tell, since most of it came out of him spontaneously, even though he didn't tell it all that first time.

Mari reported the abuse to the police and the case went to trial. There Leif was acquitted. Nicklas's story and Mari's testimony stood against Leif's denial. The court did not find proof of a crime. Nicklas started therapy at the Boys' Clinic.

Now Nicklas feels so incredibly much better, it has gone so fast. You can see it in his eyes. He has that twinkle in his eyes again, which he hasn't had for several years. It started coming back once he told. It's become so clear, he has something much softer in his eyes and he doesn't have to hug as hard as before.

22. Obstacles and problems in the treatment work

A father has confessed that he has sexually abused his son for a number of years. This is reported to both the police and the social welfare authorities. The father is sentenced to prison, placed in an institution where he is offered and accepts psychotherapy. The social services quickly investigate the needs of the other family members and assume responsibility for co-ordinating the necessary treatment interventions. This means that all family members are offered supportive conversation and therapy in various forms. A confidential openness prevails in the professional network around the family. The different professional agencies consult with each other concerning the family members' situation, needs and progress. To be able to deal with any conflicts that may arise due to the professionals in the network becoming proxies for the feelings carried by their respective clients, the social services have appointed a qualified case manager for the group.

This is a fictitious situation, a model situation we have only very rarely come close to in reality. Reality is in most cases very far from this hypothetical example. Usually the perpetrator denies his guilt and is unmotivated for treatment. Family members and friends are divided into two antagonistic camps: those who believe and those who do not believe that sexual abuse has occurred. The victim is confused and finds it increasingly difficult to figure out what has actually happened.

Marianne, a well-educated upper-class woman, financially independent, with an exclusive apartment in central Stockholm, telephoned the Clinic. She said that her son, Fredrik, four years old, had begun to do "strange things" that he had never done before. He turned up his bottom at her when he was getting ready for bed, he couldn't get to sleep, fussed when he had to go to the toilet, had begun to lose control of his bowels, "fooled around" with his penis and sometimes had a red bottom. He drew bad and nice men who sometimes became "daddy" and moved his hand back and forth in frantic gestures and said that his daddy wanted him to do that. Marianne interpreted them as masturbating movements.

Marianne believed that Fredrik was being sexually abused by his father and that he was in need of help to deal with "this horrible thing he's been through, so that he won't be harmed by it in the future". The reason she phoned Save the Children was that she didn't think at that time that she had to report her husband to the police. She "didn't think it would lead anywhere" and she didn't want to "get the social authorities mixed up in it". As it turned out, she didn't really know what "the social authorities" were.

We said that either Fredrik had been sexually abused, in which case it was difficult to help him as long as he was at risk of being subjected to further sexual abuse; or he had not been sexually abused, in which case there was no reason for him to come to the Boys' Clinic. We suggested that if she was convinced that the boy had been sexually abused, she should first go to the police and report it. The mother replied once again that she didn't want to report it and that she planned to "make sure that Fredrik wasn't left alone with his father anymore". Besides, he worked so much that he was hardly ever home. Their marriage was falling apart, but it would take time to arrange "all the practical and financial details".

She had confronted her husband with her suspicions and she had also told her sister, who was certain that Fredrik was being sexually abused. The husband denied it and said that Marianne "was out of her mind".

We met Marianne on several occasions and understood she was in a state of shock in which she wasn't capable of seeing the consequences of the various alternatives she was now faced with. She said that on the one hand if the father could not be convicted of sexual abuse, there wasn't any point in reporting the matter to the police. Fredrik would just be subjected to more painful situations, she thought. On the other hand, it wasn't good if he was convicted either. "After all, we're talking about Fredrik's father, neither Fredrik nor I have anything to gain by putting him behind bars," she said. "I don't want to put anyone in prison, I want Fredrik to get help. That's why I'm turning to you."

She could negotiate with her husband and try to get him to agree not to be alone with Fredrik, and she thought he would go along with it because he was afraid she would report him to the police otherwise. Besides, she was in a good bargaining position in the negotiations concerning the financial terms of the divorce. In other words, she thought she could "blackmail" her husband into keeping away from Fredrik in the future. We advised her that as soon as her husband got fed up with her dictating the terms in this manner, he could go to an attorney and claim that she was interfering with his visitation rights and very quickly get the court on his side. To report him for incest at that point would put her credibility in doubt, so it would be better if she reported her suspicions now.

At this early stage of the contact the focus was entirely on Marianne. We let her consult anonymously with a police officer and a social secretary who had experience with sexual abuse cases. Finally she decided to file a report, which in this case was a prerequisite for accepting Fredrik into therapy. After questioning and examination by a child psychologist, Fredrik eventually came to the Boys' Clinic for treatment.

WHEN THERE IS GOOD REASON TO BE AFRAID

Ronny had been subjected to violent sadistic abuse by his father. The father had been convicted by a court of law, despite a plea of not guilty. In such cases the children sometimes have good reason to be afraid. Among those children who have been subjected to violent and sadistic abuse by their fathers, we have experience of a few cases where the fathers have threatened to take revenge for what they claim are the false accusations to which they have been subjected by both the child and the ex-wife. Men like this may threaten to kidnap the child and beat up its mother or even kill her.

In such a situation it is impossible to start therapy to deal with the aftermath of the sexual abuse until the child feels it is safe. In such an acute phase, which can be prolonged, it is instead a question of making sure to have secure locks on the door, of determining whether the walls of the house can be climbed, of knowing whom to call in the middle of the night, how fast the police can get there and whether the father knows which school the child is attending.

In such a situation, the social services and the police must act to guarantee the family protection.

WHEN THE CHILD COMES FOR HIS MOTHER'S SAKE

Mothers of children who have been sexually abused have many difficulties to get through, whether the perpetrator is the father of the children, a close friend or relative, or an outsider. All the feelings and the anxiety caused by the abuse must often be dealt with by the mother entirely on her own. These feelings may include worry about what will happen with the child in the future, ambivalent feelings about the child's behaviour, and feelings of guilt and shame.

To add to the burden there are prolonged police investigations, drawn-out custody battles if the father is the perpetrator, divorce, the perpetrator's persistent denial, other people's disbelief, and perhaps on top of all this the mother may brood about the possibility that she herself was sexually abused as a child. Taken together, all these worries often bring the mother to the brink of a nervous breakdown.

Most mothers have enough strength and support from friends and relatives to prevent them from shifting too much of their own concern onto the child. They are able to differentiate between their own needs and those of the child. We have, however, encountered a few mothers who were not able to do this.

The child naturally senses this, and besides having to struggle with the after-effects of the abuse to which it has been subjected, the child also feels responsibility and justified concern for the welfare of the mother and is tormented by the thought that it may have been the cause of her troubles.

One way to approach this is to get the child to visit us for a period so that "mummy will be a little less worried", which she often is when we begin a therapeutic collaboration. She is no longer alone and has "experts" taking care of her boy.

The question then arises as to what the focus of the treatment should be: the mother's concern or the fears, fantasies and feelings that have to do with the abuse itself. It has been found that those boys who are most caught up in their mother's worry have the hardest time letting out their own anxiety and fear. They enter a state of denial and are uncooperative, keep looking at the clock and wonder when they're going to get to go home. In these situations it is not possible to give the child any meaningful therapy for the after-effects of the actual abuse. The focus must instead be the mother's anxiety and how the boy can relate to it.

WHEN OTHER FAMILY MEMBERS DENY AND PLAY DOWN THE ABUSE

We sometimes encounter family members who, when it is disclosed that the children have been sexually abused for several years, impatiently wonder how long it will be before "we are a real family again". It may be mothers who, shortly after the abuse has been disclosed, appeal to the children that they should feel sorry for their father and understand that "daddy has been ill and has suffered and couldn't help doing what he did".

"Even though daddy has behaved badly he is sorry now and would be very happy if you were to wish him a happy Father's Day."

Such an attitude is as difficult for the victim to relate to as the opposite, when friends and relatives make the perpetrator out to be a fiend. When such reactions occur it is particularly important that the entire family be offered support and therapy.

WHEN BOYS REMAIN SILENT

We have on a number of occasions come into contact with boys for whom the evidence is conclusive that they have been gravely sexually abused for a very long time. Some of these boys think this is nothing to talk about. Instead they want to forget what has happened and make an effort not to think about it.

These cases have often involved teenage boys who are well-known to the police and social authorities for criminality, alcohol and drug abuse, violent behaviour, abuse of other children and other symptoms that can be attributed more or less to the abuse they themselves have suffered.

They have come to us through the social services, the foster home in which they live, or because the parents feel the boy is in need of therapy. They usually agree to come see us a few times. Our offer of treatment is based on voluntary co-operation and some kind of inner motivation for change on the part of the client.

These "unmotivated" boys have developed extremely strong external defences against their problems. During the therapy sessions they have nevertheless reluctantly agreed to attend, they have been found to bear a great deal of hate and disappointment towards the adult world, with more or less explicit fantasies of violence and revenge towards those who have let them down and abused them. All of these boys have been without fathers, either because their fathers are dead or because they have disappeared for other reasons.

We are well aware of the fact that these boys are very much in the risk zone for further sexual abuse, drug and alcohol abuse, and criminality if they cannot be motivated to take part in some form of therapy. Nevertheless, we must admit that we have sometimes failed to motivate them for treatment.

WHEN SUSPECTED ABUSERS FEEL UNJUSTLY TREATED
Occasionally the social services, even though the court has acquitted the abuser of the accusation, refuse to allow the father to have unsupervised visitation with the child he is suspected of abusing. The evidence has not been sufficient for a conviction. But the child has been remitted to us for treatment due to symptoms deemed by the social services to be linked to the fact that the child must nevertheless have been subjected to sexual abuse.

These fathers feel unjustly treated, opposed at every turn and persecuted, and it has happened that they have come to us, sometimes threateningly, and accused us of taking the mother's side. "Naturally the child is unhappy when it is not allowed to see its father under natural forms", say these fathers, "and the best thing for the child would be to arrange this as soon as possible." They wonder why, if we have the best interests of the child at heart, we don't think it is as important for a child to have contact with its father as with its mother. They send long letters, independent reports, lie-detector tests etc. to prove their innocence, and so on.

When it is not compatible with our role and the therapeutic agreement we have with the child, we must turn down these fathers. As the children's therapists we cannot simultaneously help these fathers with their bitterness, disappointment and despair. They must be offered support and help from another quarter.

23. Keeping the door open on uncertainty

It happens that children take back their stories of sexual abuse. This is most common in cases of sexual abuse within the family. When a child first denies, then admits and then takes back his admission, Furniss (1991) calls this secondary denial, since it always follows an initial primary denial of abuse. Between these denials, the child gives a description of abusive events which is often very believable.

Secondary denial is one of the areas of uncertainty which all professional treatment providers and other professionals who work with child sexual abuse cases have to deal with.

The extensive media attention given to sexual abuse has increased the risk of misinterpretations and panicky reactions. It has also increased the opportunities of discovering adequate signs of sexual abuse.

A red bottom when the baby has been with its father may indicate more than the fact that the father has been remiss in changing diapers. To a mother worried about incest, it can also mean sexual abuse. A male teacher who is deeply dedicated to the children under his charge may arouse suspicions of paedophilia in concerned parents and colleagues. No one knows if there are grounds for the suspicions or not.

When children themselves do not give any verification of suspicions of sexual abuse, we naturally ask ourselves: Does the abuse exist in reality or does it only exist in the minds of worried family members? The right to remain unsure, to keep the door open on uncertainty, is something that we as treatment professionals think is important to defend.

What do we do when a parent comes to the clinic and claims that the child has been sexually abused, but the child denies it or says it doesn't remember? Should children be treated for sexual abuse they themselves cannot admit to or talk about, and in cases where there are no witnesses or any forensic evidence to back up the suspicions of abuse?

We have taken children into therapy who have not been able themselves to admit that they have been subjected to sexual abuse, but where the parents have resolutely asserted it. They have included both children where the suspicion of crime has been reported to the police but not led to prosecution, and children where the suspicion of crime has not been reported to the police.

With time we have learned that the prospects for successful therapy are not good if the child itself cannot in any way verify the parents' suspicion. We have therefore increasingly begun to meet only the parents of these "silent children". In this way we avoid putting excessive pressure on the child to force it to give information it cannot give.

However, sometimes the parent is adamant in wanting us to meet the child, at the same time as we feel that a few conversations with the child would give us a clearer picture of whether the conditions are ripe for initiating a course of therapy. Then we give the child several appointments, no more than three. If, during the sessions, the child still cannot admit in any way that it has been subjected to sexual abuse, we call off the therapy. Our conclusion is that the child either is not ready to face up to and deal with the abuse, or that none has taken place. In this situation we feel it would be wrong to continue the contact with the child.

We believe that children who are forced to attend therapy in order to alleviate the parents' anxiety lose their own motivation to seek help. We do not think that persuading a reluctant child to attend some sessions at the Boys' Clinic is harmful. But we do not want to be a part of forcing a child into a fruitless contact with us. We can, however, continue meeting the worried parent.

MOTHER CONVINCED

We will now consider two cases which illustrate in different ways the

146

discussion regarding certain and uncertain. The first case involves a mother who was certain that her son was sexually abused, whereas the son was not as convinced.

Erik, twelve years old, came to us with his mother. The mother said that Erik had been sexually abused by his grandfather. Erik said that he couldn't recall being abused.

During her own childhood as well as Erik's, the mother had often been ill. She had been confined to bed for long periods with severe anxiety and somatic symptoms such as the feeling that she couldn't breathe and that her legs wouldn't carry her.

When the mother began in therapy as an adult, she got in touch with memories from her child and adolescent years: her father had sexually abused her. She then broke off contact with her parents. After some time she wrote a letter to her father and explained why she didn't want to see him anymore. He didn't reply to the letter, but sent a check for SEK 20,000. She regarded the money as a tacit admission and an attempt at compensation from her father.

Erik was very interested in sports. But he had developed a somewhat cautious and timid attitude towards others. He never quarrelled with his mother, who was so fragile and sickly. He spent a lot of time in his room playing video games. Erik had symptoms that troubled him. He had frequent stomachaches and inexplicable coughing fits, as if something were caught in his throat that he had to cough up.

Erik had spent several summers with his grandparents. When his mother became aware that she had been sexually abused by her own father she became doubly terrified. Had grandpa done anything sexual with her Erik as well? He had been there every summer. The stomachaches and the coughing fits, which were reminiscent of her own symptoms | were they signs of sexual abuse by Erik's grandfather? Suddenly it became clear to the mother that Erik had also been sexually abused. The mother couldn't rest until Erik told her about the abuse.

ALLEVIATE MOTHER'S ANXIETY

Now Erik had another problem to deal with. He could only alleviate his mother's anxiety by telling her he had been sexually abused by his grandfather. But he couldn't remember any abuse. Should he tell her that something happened even though he couldn't remember it happening and even though it may not have happened just to calm his mother?

Erik was asked:

"Think of a scale from one to ten. Ten means you're completely sure that you were sexually abused by your grandpa. One means you're completely sure that you haven't been sexually abused by your grandpa. What number do you choose?"

"Five," said Erik.

When asked why he had picked five, Erik replied that it was because his mother believed his grandfather had sexually abused him. The therapist asked what number he would choose if he disregarded what his mother believed.

"Two," said Erik.

When Erik explained what the two points consisted of, he said one point was for the pain in his stomach and the other was for his coughing problems. He had no memories or fragments of memories regarding any sexual abuse.

Our contact with Erik was terminated, but our contact with his mother continued for several sessions. We did not question her conviction that Erik had been sexually abused by his grandfather. Nor did we confirm it. We did, however, point out the fact that she herself had needed time before she could remember what she had been through. It was possible that Erik also needed time, perhaps several years, before he would be motivated to dig into his own memories. We also pointed out the possibility that Erik may not have been sexually abused at all.

SEVERAL POSSIBILITIES OPEN

Our other example has to do with being able to handle the uncertainty in the actual treatment.

Jesper, twelve years old, was the eldest of three siblings. His father had been sentenced to prison for sexual abuse of Jesper's middle sister, who was seven years old.

She had told their mother that daddy had poked her in the fanny while she was sleeping so that she had woken up and cried because it had hurt

148

and that daddy had pressed his willy against her crack.

A medical examination revealed that she had scar tissue from tear wounds around her vaginal opening and damage to her hymen.

Jesper was deeply depressed and had suicidal thoughts. He blamed himself for his father's conviction. Both Jesper and his little sister were offered treatment at the Boys' Clinic. The youngest sister had been with her grandmother and was not involved in any way.

The children had been interrogated by the police. Jesper's sister stuck to her story and said that Jesper had also woken up when she was sad, seen what daddy had done and consoled her when daddy got up and made porridge.

Jesper was interrogated by the police on several occasions but stubbornly denied having seen anything strange going on between his father and his little sister. He remembered when it was supposed to have happened, the father and the children were on a holiday trip and living in a rented house on the Mediterranean.

In one police interrogation he remembered "a little", that he had been woken up by his little sister's crying, that he had consoled her and that daddy had then brought porridge. During the next interrogation he remembered that he had seen daddy "poke" his little sister, but not really where and eventually he had told under great stress and many tears pretty much exactly the same story as his little sister. Afterwards he was greatly relieved.

Then two months passed before he told his mother that he was so unhappy because he had lied to the police, that he had done it so he would not have to go there anymore. He thought that if he told them what he thought they wanted to hear they would be satisfied.

In this situation, we as therapists are of course unable to know what is true and what isn't. We cannot tell by looking at the boy whether he is telling the truth or not. What we can do is to bear in mind that it is not unusual for children to take back their stories in this manner. Furthermore, we can check to see whether his and his little sister's versions agree in detail. It isn't really our job to ferret out the truth in this situation, but to listen and acknowledge Jesper's misery at the situation in which he finds himself.

The therapist said to Jesper:

"Only you yourself know, deep inside, what you have seen or not seen, what has happened or not happened. I have no way of knowing. All I know with certainty is that a boy like you with all his heart does not want to accept that a thing like this happens in his family." Then Jesper started to weep uncontrollably, while nodding his head almost unnoticeably.

He missed his father deeply. He didn't want to accept the thought that his father had sexually abused his little sister. "I feel sorry for my daddy who isn't allowed to meet his children. He misses us." His father had been a very strong presence in the children's lives and his loss was extremely palpable when they weren't allowed to see him and he might end up going to prison. Did Jesper perhaps believe that by retracting his story he would get his father back?

In our contact with Jesper it was important to show him that this could be one possibility. At the same time we naturally had to be open to the other possibility, that he had made up what he said to get out of going to the police. This uncertainty regarding what was true or false, dealt with in this manner, did not prove to be any obstacle to initiating a course of therapy with Jesper.

CERTAINTY IN MOST CASES

Being allowed to be unsure when we don't know is important for us. It doesn't mean that we never know. Usually what children have told us is so unambiguous that we feel certain that they have been sexually abused. This certainty exists even in many of the cases where charges have not been brought or where the perpetrator has been acquitted by a court of law. Most children who have come to us have been able to describe, draw and express details of the abuse which our experience has shown indicate that it must have happened. And most parents who have come to us have allowed their children the space and time they needed to process their difficult experiences at their own speed.

It is not the group of children and parents we have discussed here, but rather a much smaller group, where the children have been unable to tell. The problems are naturally greater in the case of pre-school children who are unable to describe the abuse themselves.

But we believe that our fundamental rule of keeping the door open on our own uncertainty in unclear cases has given us a therapeutic platform which has proved to be fruitful.

24. Being surprised by our own feelings

Naturally children's feelings, both those that are expressed and those that have been suppressed, affect our own feelings and fantasies. Observing and reflecting on our own emotions aroused in therapy is one of our most important sources of information on the patient (Holm 1987). This well-known process is called counter-transference.

The basic idea of the counter-transference concept is that the feelings aroused in the therapist reflect a subconscious sympathy for the processes taking place in the patient, that these reactions are not immediately conscious, but that they can be discovered through the therapist's own associations during therapy (Sandler et al. 1973). These subconscious feelings on the part of the therapist can be used as a tool to understand the client. But does counter-transference really have to do with the client, or do the emotions we feel during therapy mainly have to do with ourselves and our own past lives? Making this distinction requires self-knowledge and guidance.

In our meetings with the children at the Boys' Clinic, we have experienced strong and extreme feelings that have sometimes been understandable, sometimes enigmatic, sometimes frightening and painful. These feelings haven't only had to do with us and the individual client, but also with the whole problem complex surrounding sexual abuse. The counter-transference reactions we have had and which we describe here below are feelings which anyone who comes into close contact with sexually abused children is likely to experience.

AVENGER FEELING

One of the first strong feelings we experienced when we encountered several sexually abused boys where the perpetrator had got off without prosecution or punishment was a primitive lust for revenge. We started fantasizing about opening a secret branch of the Boys' Clinic which was devoted to night-time vigilante activities aimed at liquidating these monstrous child abusers which the justice system failed to deal with.

This "avenger feeling" was from the start more an expression of our own frustration than an indication of the children's feelings toward their abusers. The more children we have met, the more we have been impressed by the ambivalence of the children's feelings. They both love and hate, long for and want to flee from their abusers. The more aware we became of the children's complex and contradictory feelings toward their abusers, the more our own avenger feelings diminished.

But they have returned at times, especially when we have encountered children who have been sadistically abused by perpetrators for whom they have felt purer emotions of fear and hatred. Due to the great number of children we have worked with, this avenger feeling has developed into a useful counter-transference reaction that gives us an indication that the child may have very strong feelings of fear and rage and very weak, if any, feelings of longing and love for the perpetrator.

DETECTIVE FEELING

Sometimes we have been faced with stories, information and circumstances that we have had difficulty interpreting. Examples are mothers who have told us that their child has been sexually abused, usually by the child's father, whereas the child has said nothing or very little to us that confirms the mother's story. Our uncertainty has increased when the parent has given us drawings done by the child at home which the parent has one-sidedly interpreted as expressions of sexual abuse, but where we have not been as certain.

In our contact with these "silent" children and in our inter-professional consultations on these cases we have felt a strong desire to change profession and become private detectives. We have fantasized about investigating the man under suspicion in the minutest detail, equipped

154

with bugging devices and night-vision binoculars, shadowing him every minute of the day. The need to know has sometimes been so great that we have fantasized about installing assault alarms and secret video cameras in the children's bedrooms to either catch the suspected perpetrator in flagrante delicto or prove that the mother's story isn't true.

This "detective feeling" has taught us how important it is to be able to handle uncertainty in work with sexually abused children. As we noted earlier, we must be able to cope with not knowing exactly what has happened and sometimes we must be able to live with not knowing if any sexual abuse has occurred at all.

Not allowing ourselves to feel sure until we have been completely convinced has been difficult, especially when the pressure on us from the accusing parent has been strong. Questioning a mother's reliability can be tantamount in her eyes to not believing the child. The fact that the child has not said anything to us is then something we must vigilantly bear in mind.

As a counter-transference reaction, the detective feeling can indicate a confusion on the part of the child as to what has happened. The detective feeling has helped us to understand that it is extra important in these cases to give the child his own space in therapy.

FEELING OF POWERLESSNESS AND UNREALITY

When mother's stories about what their children have been through have had to do with ritual abuse, satanic sects, cannibalism, burials, crucifixions, ritual child murders, acts such as drinking blood and eating eyes, mutilations etc., the detective feeling has been supplanted by a feeling of unreality.

With each visit to the clinic, the stories have become embroidered with increasingly incredible details. Is this mother crazy, or is it we who are not capable of facing the possibility of ritual and satanic abuse?

When the child has failed in either word or deed to confirm the horrible stories told by the mothers, the feeling of powerlessness has increased. Isn't this a case of a mentally ill mother who is projecting her own fantasies onto the child? Can they be unprocessed traumatic reactions stemming from abuse she herself was once a victim of, now projected onto the child?

In these cases as well, we have found it best to try to accept not knowing, to resist dismissing what may seem to us to be outrageous fantasies. We cannot know whether these extreme stories are true, partially true or false. And even if the stories are not true, the child still has a real problem it needs help with: a mother with serious psychological problems.

But we have also experienced feelings of unreality for quite different reasons:

"I know that my daddy will get out of prison in two years. Then I'll be nine years old and then I think he's going to kill me and my little brother. First he'll come to school and pick us up so that mummy doesn't have a chance to phone the police."

These are the words of a seven-year-old boy whose father was in prison for both murder and attempted murder, and for sexual abuse of his children. He said it sort of in passing, without emotion, on his way to the therapy room.

The implications of such a statement, the boundless terror and despair which this expresses – notwithstanding the detached tone – is very difficult to comprehend and empathize with.

There is a tendency for the therapist to assume the same detached attitude and say something along the lines of: "We don't really believe that, do we?" or "I'm sure he won't do that." The counter-transference feeling of unreality on the part of the therapist tells us something about the child's efforts to cope and come to terms with an intolerable situation and helps us to understand something of what is going on inside the child's head. In this case the therapist was able to take guidance from his own feeling of unreality and instead say: "You're brave to tell me such a scary thing as that. How horrible to be afraid of being killed by your own father."

ABUSER FEELING

We stress the importance of having the child describe the abuse in detail in therapy. Sexual abuse is just that: sexual. Sometimes it feels as if we ourselves have repeated the abuse when we try to get the children to tell us what they have been through. We have felt like "dirty old men" talking dirty with children.

156

It's a difficult feeling to deal with. Many of the children have been sexually abused by men in situations similar to that in which the child finds himself at the Boys' Clinic: alone in a room with an adult man, where his mother can't see what's going on. The experience of that feeling has sometimes made the therapist double-check to make sure he has his fly zipped, clean hands, whether he has stains on his clothes, whether his shirttail is hanging out, and so forth. When this feeling has been strong, the therapist has also felt the need to maintain a physical distance from the child.

As a counter-transference reaction, the "abuser feeling" can tell us about the child's feeling of vulnerability and helplessness. The abuser feeling has made us aware of how important it is to respect the sexually abused child's boundaries and integrity, not to invade the child with our questions, to first ask if it is OK if we ask, and not to be misled by the child's inability to say no, springing from a need to please others.

INCOMPETENCE FEELING

Now and then we have experienced the feeling of being incompetent as treatment providers. Instead of providing treatment, we have felt as if we were merely minding the children while the mothers sat in the waiting room reading magazines. The children have been interested in everything but the purpose of the visit.

The feeling of being incompetent may have to do with our eagerness and our ambition to be successful, effective and able therapists. Perhaps the children who didn't want to be treated were trying to tell us that we were moving too fast and that they didn't feel enough trust and confidence to dare to approach what they had come for.

"I just want to play and you should be quiet and just talk if I ask you about something," said one seven-year-old boy, who for a long period of time did not want to answer any questions about sexual abuse.

The feeling of being incompetent may also tell us that the child is, for other reasons, not ready to open up for treatment. The underlying reason may be threats, magical notions of punishment, or a desire to reunite the family.

Sometimes we have encountered boys who have been let down by everyone around them at all levels. Children who have had to put up with being invisible to the adults around them, who have been subjected to repeated abuse, perhaps placed in unsuitable foster homes, transferred to another foster home and finally taken back home again by a periodically alcohol-abusing father. In other words, children who have gone from one wretched situation to another.

That is when the adoption feeling can arise. We get the urge to take the boy in our arms, take him home with us, draw a hot bath for him and give him a nice big cup of steaming hot chocolate afterwards. And finally tuck him into bed, read him fairy-tales and protect him against all evil until he grows up!

Not all children who have been let down and had a very rough time have given us these adoption feelings. It is the children who, despite all the wretchedness they have been through, have not lost their ability to relate, have not isolated themselves in acting-out behaviour and impenetrable defences. Children who have remained to some extent reachable and able to form an attachment to us.

This counter-transference reaction can thereby tell us that the child may have also had something positive in its life that we have overlooked, that perhaps it has been given a certain measure of care and love so that this ability to relate positively and form attachments has been preserved. Accordingly, the adoption feeling may indicate that there is more to discover, that there may be significant persons who have given the child relatively secure periods. Persons who, with help and encouragement, may be able to re-establish a positive relationship.

The adoption feeling may also tell us something about the times we ourselves have been let down, and it may be a way of dealing with a feeling of abandonment we ourselves carry within us. This is important to be aware of and to keep separate from the therapy work.

25. Concluding discussion

Sexually abused boys need to be given an opportunity to express their feelings about what they have been through. A sexually abused boy is at risk of abusing others himself. The root of the problem lies in unprocessed feelings of fear, shame, denied grief and oppression, which in the emotionally abandoned child risk being transformed into their opposites. The rage that springs from the denied feelings is a breeding ground for perversion. The childhood trauma can be turned into destructive triumph (see Chapters 3, 12 and 16).

Unfortunately, we have not always been able to get sexually abused boys to express their feelings regarding themselves as victims, even though they have come to the Boys' Clinic voluntarily and even though we have known what they have been through. We have not been able to motivate some of these boys to remain in therapy, especially some of the teenagers we have been in contact with. We think this is a problem, since they need to process what they have been through, otherwise there is a risk they will themselves commit sexual abuse or other kinds of violent crime (see Chapter 22).

RISK OF NEW ABUSE

Watkins and Bentovim (1992) believe that there is a significant risk that a sexually abused boy will sexually abuse others. Based on a review of three studies, the two researchers estimate that one of five sexually abused boys themselves abuse others. According to them, sexual abuse is the fourth most common symptom exhibited by sexually abused boys.

Glasgow et al. (1994) report the results of a study conducted in Liverpool. It shows that one-third of all those who were accused of sexual abuse during a period of one year were seventeen years old or younger. The same article presents the results of a couple of studies where over fifty percent of the sexual offenders started their career in sexual crime as teenagers. The National Children's Home (1992) published a report commissioned by the Department of Health that confirms the Liverpool study. Here as well, one-third of the sexual offenders were young.

It is during adolescence that deviant behaviours begin to manifest themselves in the form of serious offences. If these young people are not taken in tow then, or preferably even earlier, there is a risk that they will continue into adult life as sex offenders. When we set aside resources for the treatment of sexually abused boys, we not only help the individual child, we also reduce the risk that the children of the next generation will be subjected to sexual abuse.

The fact that we sometimes fail in our ambitions to help sexually abused teenage boys shows how urgent it is to improve the treatment methods.

DIFFERENCES BETWEEN BOYS AND GIRLS

What is the difference between being sexually abused as a boy and as a girl? As far as suffering and physical and mental damage, it is of course not possible to measure the differences in terms of who suffers the most. But there are differences between how boys and girls handle painful events. Sexually abused boys run a much greater risk of becoming abusers themselves than do girls.

Finkelhor (1986) reflects over what the reason might be that women don't abuse children to the same extent as men. According to Finkelhor, women are:

- less dependent on being dominant in sexual relationships
- less inclined to have casual or several simultaneous sexual relationships
- less inclined to view sex in isolation from other feelings for the partner
- less affected, in terms of self-esteem, if they are temporarily not in a sexual relationship

- more empathetic to children's needs.

In the above-cited literature review, Watkins and Bentovim made a systematic comparison between boys and girls with regard to sexual abuse. Based on these studies they developed the following hypotheses.

Sexually abused boys, compared to sexually abused girls, are:

- younger
- more often physically abused as well
- more often abused forcefully
- less often alone when the abuse takes place
- less willing to tell
- more often physically injured
- more often subjected to masturbatory abuse
- more often subjected to orogenital abuse
- more often subjected to anal abuse
- less often subjected to non-contact abuse

Perpetrators who abuse boys sexually are:

- more often extrafamilial
- more often strangers
- more often adolescents
- more often involved in a sex ring
- more often fathers than stepfathers
- more often professionals who work with children
- if the perpetrator is female, it is more likely that she abuses boys than girls

Society's response on behalf of sexually abused boys:

- involves police more often
- recognizes less need for protection
- recognizes less need for separation from family
- provides less treatment

Nothing in our work with sexually abused boys refutes these hypotheses.

PAEDOPHILIC ABUSE

Victims of sexual abuse committed by child care professionals have proved to be a large group in our therapy. We discuss paedophilic abuse in Chapters 6, 18 and 19. Approximately one-quarter of the victims we have treated have been sexually abused by teachers, youth recreation leaders, contact persons appointed by the social services, day nursery staff, etc. Naturally, this type of abuse is a small problem, in terms of scope, compared with many other problems in society. Yet it is alarming that our children risk being sexually abused by professionals within the institutions that are supposed to provide for their care, welfare and education. There are female paedophiles, but the vast majority are men. Of the children that have come to the Boys' Clinic for sexual abuse by paedophiles, all have been victimized by male abusers. At the same time it is important that adult men work with children. Boys must be exposed to good male role models.

BACKGROUND CHECK

Is it possible to identify the few male paedophile risk persons who work with children? There must naturally be a limit to how much an employer is entitled to find out about a job applicant. This limit varies in different professions. Background checks are required for taxi drivers in Stockholm nowadays to check for any criminal record. They are denied licences to operate a taxi if they have previously been convicted of a violent crime. Would it be possible to require background checks on people who work with children? Are the relatively small risks a child runs of being sexually abused by a male staff member at a day nursery, by a male teacher in school, or by a male sports coach, comparable to the relatively small risk a passenger in a taxi runs of being assaulted by the driver? If so, why are background checks run on professionals who primarily work with the transport of adults, but not on those who work with the care of children?

PREVENTION

The safety of children is naturally not solely a question of reliable personnel. We Swedes consider ourselves world leaders in child safety in a number of respects. When it comes to helmets, car seats, school crossing guards and swimming skills, we seem to be in agreement on how urgent this safety-mindedness is. Prevention, information, education and campaigns are necessary and universally accepted in these contexts.

When it comes to protecting children against sexual abuse, however, we are more cautious and less sure of ourselves. What do we say to the children? How do we explain to children that there are adults who want to do sexual things with children, even within the family? Doesn't it just frighten and worry them unnecessarily if we start putting books in their hands, show films or try in other ways to explain these complicated matters to them? The question of how to approach the subject of sexual abuse with children does indeed involve some difficult judgements.

By its very nature, sexual abuse is connected with secrecy. We believe that the openness displayed by the media in this field in recent years is for the most part beneficial. Newspaper articles and television programmes on the topic have helped adults to realize that boys can also be victims of sexual abuse. But this openness has also had other effects. Not infrequently, a boy's visit to the Boys' Clinic has been precipitated by an article he has read in the paper or a programme he has seen on TV about sexual abuse, after which he has told one of his parents that he has been abused himself.

THE FAMILY PERSPECTIVE

Approximately half of the children we have had in therapy have been sexually abused within the family. Not always by parents, sometimes by siblings, but most have been abused by their biological fathers.

Intrafamilial sexual abuse can be difficult to disclose. The child's dependence on his parents, fear of what will happen if the abuse is discovered, shame, and loyalty towards the abusing parent reduce the likelihood that these crimes will be revealed.

Sexually abused children may suffer from stomachaches and an inability to concentrate, they may display sexualized behaviour, they may be self-destructive, detached, etc. But these symptoms may also be displayed by children who have not been sexually abused. We have not found any typical abuse syndrome or a pattern of symptoms that indicates with certainty that a child has been subjected to sexual abuse.

The children that have come to us and have been sexually abused in

163

the home have either spontaneously told an adult close to them, usually the mother, or else some adult has suspected abuse and asked the child, again usually the mother.

In those cases where the biological mothers have been the abusers, the boys have not dared to disclose the abuse. Only after heavy pressure from other concerned persons close to the child have these children admitted to abuse by their mothers, who have then confessed.

Sibling abuse has usually been revealed by one of the siblings, usually the younger, telling one of the parents.

For the same reasons that intrafamilial abuse is more difficult to disclose than extrafamilial abuse, it is also more difficult to treat. The road back to a more or less normal life is longer for children who have been abused within the home.

The boys we have had in therapy who have been sexually abused by a parent have generally not only lost contact with the abusing parent, but also with relatives on the abuser's side. Many of these boys have harboured a more or less secret longing for their lost parent. It is naturally not the abusive side of the parent they have longed for, but "the nice" parent. The child's ambivalent feelings for the abuser are a reality which cannot be neglected when it comes to intrafamilial abuse (see Chapter 16).

It is important to affirm the need of children to put painful events behind them and live a normal life. It may feel more abnormal for a sexually abused boy to talk to his classmates about a father he never meets than to talk about a father he meets sometimes in the company of a third person.

We ourselves think that we have sometimes been too passive in communicating the need of sexually abused boys to have some sort of contact with the abusing parent.

The same applies to those relatives that have found themselves in conflict with the non-abusing parent as a result of the abuse. The conflicts have often arisen when the parents of a denying abuser take the side of the abuser. This has led to a break in contact with the grandchild, which can be very unfortunate for all parties.

To a greater extent than before, we now explore the feasibility of allowing the boy to meet the abusing parent under safe forms, in other words where there is no risk of further abuse. This assumes he wants to do so himself and also requires a thorough discussion with the boy about his expectations and feelings for such a meeting. It is naturally positive if the abuser himself has owned up to and assumed responsibility for the abuse, but it cannot be the only criterion for whether a child who wishes to meet the abusing parent should be allowed to or not.

Taking the family approach when children are in need of psychotherapy has been a firmly established principle for a long time now. Family therapy and network interventions are common techniques included in most treatment contexts. But in the case of sexual abuse, nothing should be taken for granted. No matter how the problem is approached, problems arise. Traditional family therapy sessions can be difficult and in some cases directly unsuitable. Including a denying abuser in a family therapy session can be so difficult for the child that it refuses to say anything or even takes back what it has said previously. In the case of sexually abused children, it may be necessary to limit therapy sessions to parts of the family and the network for a period of time. This makes it all the more important not to lose the family perspective.

At the Boys' Clinic we have participated in professional networks around families in which incest has occurred. In one case the father had been convicted of sexual abuse. He received psychotherapy at the correctional institution. The children had one therapist, the mother another. A home therapist was available at times to support the mother and children in the home environment.

There is a risk in adopting this kind of interprofessional treatment model, namely that the different therapists will be inundated with "their" patient's feelings and become caught up in them so that the family's conflicts are transferred to and mirrored in the therapeutic system. Through the years we have seen many examples of experienced therapists and professionals becoming involved in conflicts when working with incest families. That is why we have suggested the appointment of a co-ordinator to help in dealing with these conflicts.

When we have been involved in professional networks around an incest family, the network has met approximately five times a year for the duration of the treatment – more frequently in the beginning and less frequently towards the end. The purpose of the interprofessional efforts has not been to get the incest family back together. This has been an entirely open question which must be addressed by the family members themselves. Instead the aim has been to oppose the conspiring forces of secrecy and destructive dependence that have made the sexual abuse possible in the first place.

TREATMENT OF ABUSERS FOR CHILDREN'S SAKE

Most perpetrators of sexual abuse of children deny all or part of the crime. It would seem logical to assume that denying abusers would not accept offers of therapy. Paradoxically enough this is not always so. At the correctional institutions in Sweden which offer therapy, the abusers often initially deny their crimes. There seems to be a conflict in many of the perpetrators between denial and the need to tell and get help. But even if the abusers do not want therapy and even if some abusers who receive therapy can relapse into crime, it is important for the children's sake that they be offered qualified care and treatment during their imprisonment.

Children who have a close emotional relationship with the abuser and who are contemplating whether they should disclose the abuse are relieved if an adult informs them that the abuser will be able to get help for the "disease" that makes him subject children to sexual abuse. This is particularly true in the case of incest families – putting its father in prison where he cannot get any help, only punishment, is a heavy burden for a child to bear.

The fact that the perpetrators are in need of treatment is evident from Ulla-Britt Strömberg's (1994) interview with a psychotherapist who works with sexual offenders in prisons. "There is a strong 'consolation component' in the abuse perpetrated by an incest offender. As an adult he uses his child victims to obtain the consolation he got from masturbation when he was young. Often he imagines that the child he is abusing is living in a similar, vulnerable situation as he himself did as a child and that the child also obtains consolation from the sexual act." The interviewed therapist says that it is therefore an important theme in the therapeutic work that the abuser should understand the true implications of the abuse.

166

The Swedish Parliament has decreed that persons sentenced to prison for sexual abuse and/or physical abuse should be able to obtain treatment during their incarceration.

When this goal has been fully realized, it will be slightly less difficult to speak with children about sexual abuse.

THE UNIVERSAL AND THE UNIQUE

Psychotherapeutic work with sexually abused boys is a relatively new field of endeavour. There is still a great need to acquire knowledge regarding therapy, effects of therapy, the relationship between trauma and symptoms, which clients run the risk of abusing again, prevention and its effects, and finding investigation methods that reduce disagreement concerning the real scope of the problem.

In our work at the Boys' Clinic, we have tried to find patterns that interlink victims who have been sexually abused by their fathers, by paedophiles, by biological mothers or by siblings. The more boys we have treated, the easier it has been to see the general patterns, but at the same time the number of exceptions to the rule has grown. Why didn't the seven-year-old suffer post-traumatic syndrome after having been raped in the park by a stranger when the ten-year-old who was raped in a doorway developed many pronounced symptoms due to the assault?

Only by reflecting over these similarities and dissimilarities and the contrast between the universal and the unique, do we learn to be prepared for the fact that each new case may not conform to our expectations.

We have often experienced our clinical work as a constant learning process, where each day brings new lessons and new insights, and where our clients are our teachers. One such lesson was taught to us by nine-year-old Erik, who during one period was constantly taking trips in a time machine he built. Together with the therapist he would set off for the age of knights and chivalry, the age of dinosaurs or the space age. When they were deciding which age to travel to, the therapist and Erik would have endless discussions concerning the different dangers that threatened the different fantasy worlds. At one point, in response to Erik's direct question as to which age they should travel to this time, the therapist said:

"We'll go where you feel certain of being able to cope with the dangers that lurk there, more certain than you do in the real world. And let's hope that you will eventually be just as good at battling the dangers of the real world as you are in the time machine."

To which the boy answered: "Good, you're learning."

Bibliography

Allen, C.M. (1990): "Woman as perpertrators of child sexual abuse". I: Horton, A.L. m fl (red.), *The Incest Perpetrator – A family member no one wants to treat*. Sage Publications. USA.

Cullberg, J. (1975): *Kris och utveckling*. Natur och Kultur. Stockholm.

Edgardh, K. (1992): *SAM 73–90, Tonåringar, sex och samlevnad*. Förlagshuset Gothia AB. Göteborg.

Fairbairn, R.D. (1952): *Psychoanalytic Studies of the Personality*. Routledge. London.

Finkelhor, D. (1986): *A Sourcebook on Child Sexual Abuse. Prevention: A review of programs research*. Sage Publications. London.

Furniss, T. (1991): *The Multiprofessional Handbook of Child Sexual Abuse. Integrated management, therapy, and legal intervention*. Routledge. London.

Glasgow, D. m fl (1994): "Evidence, Incidence, Gender and Age in Sexual Abuse of Children Perpertrated by Children". I: *Child Abuse Review*, Vol.3, 1994. Wiley. Chichester.

Glasser, M. (1988): "Psychodynamic Aspects of Paedophilia". I: *Psychoanalytic Psychotherapy*, Vol. 3, nr 2, 1988, s. 121–135. Association for psychoanalytic psychotherapy in the National Health Service. London.

Hedlund, E. (1989): *Med könet som vapen och värn*. SESAM. Stockholm.

Hertoft, P. (1977): *Klinisk sexologi.* Natur och Kultur. Stockholm.

Holm, U. (1987): *Empati – att förstå andra människors känslor.* Natur och Kultur. Stockholm.

Hunter, M. (1990): *Abused Boys.* Lexington Books. New York.

Ikonen, P. & Rechardt, E. (1993): "The Origin of Shame and its Vicissitudes". I: *Scandinavian Psychoanalytic review,* nr. 16, 1993, s. 100–124. Universitetsforlaget. Oslo.

James, B. (1989): *Treating Traumatized Children.* Lexington Books. New York.

Kjellqvist, E-B. (1993): *Rött och Vitt, om skam och skamlöshet.* Carlssons Bokförlag. Stockholm.

Künstlicher, R. (1991): "Skam och ondska, om en växelverkan". I: *Vår Lösen,* nr. 5–6, 1991.

Lindbom-Jacobson, M. & Lindgren, L (1994): "Förövarens psykologi – med utgångspunkt från filmen "Music Box" av Costa Gavras". *I Psykisk Hälsa,* nr. 1, 1994.

Mangs, K. & Martell, B. (1990): *0–20 år i ett psykoanalytiskt perspektiv.* Studentlitteratur. Lund.

Martens, P. (1990): Sexualbrott mot barn, beskrivning av de misstänkta brotten. *BRÅ-rapport 1990:6.* Allmänna Förlaget. Stockholm.

Martens, P. (1991): Sexualbrott mot barn, de misstänkta förövarna. *BRÅ-rapport 1991:1.* Allmänna Förlaget. Stockholm.

Miller, A. (1993): *I begynnelsen var uppfostran.* Wahlström & Widstrand. Stockholm.

National Children's Home (1992): *Report of the Comittee of Enquiry into Children and Young People who Sexually Abuse Other Children.* National Children's Home, Central Office. London.

O'Grady, R. (1992): *För nöjes skull.* Lutherhjälpen, Rädda Barnen och Svenska kyrkans mission. Falun.

Pierce, L.H. & Pierce, R.L. (1990): "Adolescent/Sibling Incest Perpetrators". I: Horton, A.L. m fl (red.), *The Incest Perpetrator – A family member no one wants to treat.* Sage Publications. USA.

Rogers, C. & Terry, T. (1984): "Clinical Intervention with Boy Victims of Sexual Abuse. I": Stuart, I.R. & Greer, J.G. (red.), *Victims of Sexual Aggression: Treatment of Children, Women, and Men.* Van Nostrand Reinhold. New York

Salzberger-Wittenberg, I. (1993): *Psycho-Analytic Insight and Relationships, A Kleinian Approach.* Routledge. London.

Sandler, D. m fl (1973): *Grundbegreppen inom psykoanalysen. Från Freud till den moderna jagpsykologin.* Prisma. Stockholm.

Stoller, R. (1986): *The Erotic Form of Hatred.* Pantheon Books. New York.

Strömberg, U. (1994): "Forensisk psykologi: Psykoterapi med sexual-brottslingar". *Psykologtidningen*, nr. 22, 1994. Sveriges Psykologförbund.

Watkins, B. & Bentovim, A. (1992): "The Sexual Abuse of Male Children and Adolescents: A Review of Current Research". *Journal of Child Psychology and Child Psychiatry*, Vol. 33, nr. 1, 1992.

FICTION

Fölster, K. (1992): *De tre löven.* Bonniers. Stockholm.

Högberg, B. & Hesslind, L. (1979): *Kontringen.* Författarförlaget. Stockholm.

Lidman, S. (1988): *Ett herrans liv.* Wahlström & Widstrand. Stockholm.

Lundell, U. (1992): *Saknaden.* Wahlström & Widstrand. Stockholm.